Julie,
I really enjoyed
the truth of this
book. The positive tools
have been so helpful
to encourage one to press on !
Love to you all
Jeremy & Cherryl Eadon

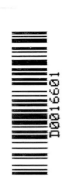
D0016601

Climb
Back
from
Cancer

ABOUT THE COVERS

The images of the two figures in silhouette on the front and back dust jacket covers of this book are not drawings, but actually digitally altered photographs of Cecilia and Alan climbing the world's largest glacial erratic (rock carried by a glacier) three years after his diagnosis. The original photographs were taken atop "Big Rock" at sunset near Okotoks, Alberta, about 25 miles south of Calgary. In a curious coincidence, on the warm spring evening on which the images were taken, the sun happened to set directly behind and along the edge of the 30 foot tall, 18,000 ton boulder. This only happens once a year and for such a photograph to be taken, perfect weather and timing are required.

Photos: Brad Wrobleski   Design: Gary Hewitt

ALSO BY ALAN HOBSON

From Everest to Enlightenment
An Adventure of the Soul

ISBN 0-9685263-0-6

The Triumph of Tenacity (formerly titled, *The Power of Passion*)
What It Takes to Get to the Top

(with co-author, Jamie Clarke) ISBN 0-9685263-3-0

Above the Bottom Line
Building Business Success through Individual Growth

(with primary author, J. Michael Fuller) ISBN 0-7715-9360-0

One Step Beyond
Rediscovering the Adventure Attitude

(with producer, John Amatt) ISBN 0-9685263-2-2

Share the Flame
The Official Retrospective Book of the [1988] Olympic Torch Relay

ISBN 0-921061-15-3

From Everest to Enlightenment, The Triumph of Tenacity
and *One Step Beyond* may be obtained by visiting
www.alanhobson.com, or for bulk orders only, by contacting:

Climb Back Inc.
#5 – 100 Prospect Heights,
Canmore, Alberta, Canada
T1W 2X8
Tel: (403) 609-9939
Fax: (403) 609-2818
info@alanhobson.com

Above the Bottom Line may be obtained by contacting:

J. Michael Fuller
Canmore, Alberta, Canada
(403) 609-4410
mfuller@telusplanet.net

WHY PAY RETAIL?

This and other books by Alan Hobson are available at substantial discounts for bulk purchases. They make ideal gifts for employees, associates, suppliers and clients; sales promotion items; premiums; fundraising vehicles; and educational tools. Special editions can also be created to meet specific needs.

For more information contact:

Climb Back Inc.
info@alanhobson.com
or
(403) 609-9939, ext. 1 (Cecilia Hobson)

CLIMB BACK

from

CANCER

Cecilia
HOBSON
AND **Alan**
HOBSON

Mt. Everest Climber
& Summiteer

Cancer Survivor

A Survivor
and Caregiver's
Inspirational
Journey

Climb Back Inc.

Copyright © 2004 Alan Hobson and Cecilia Hobson
Photographs copyright Alan Hobson and Cecilia Hobson except by permission, credits as noted.

Front cover, back cover and inside dust jacket:
Photographer: Brad Wrobleski/Cirque Dynamics, Cochrane, Alberta, Canada
www.wrobleski.com

Designer: Gary Hewitt, Wedge.a&d, Calgary, Alberta, Canada
www.visualtribe.com/wedge

This book uses American English spellings except for Canadian place names, titles, etc.

All rights reserved under International and Pan-American Copyright Conventions. No part of this book may be reproduced in any form, or by any means, electronic or mechanical, without permission in writing from the publisher, except by a reviewer, who may quote brief passages in a review to print in a magazine or newspaper or broadcast on radio, television, or the internet. Adventrepreneur is a trademark owned by Alan Hobson and Jamie Clarke. CAN/WILL® is a registered trademark owned by Alan Hobson.

Published by:

Climb Back Inc.
#5 – 100 Prospect Heights,
Canmore, Alberta, Canada
T1W 2X8

Tel: (403) 609-9939
Fax: (403) 609-2818
info@alanhobson.com
www.alanhobson.com

National Library of Canada Cataloguing in Publication

Hobson, Alan, 1958-
Climb back from cancer : a survivor and caregiver's inspirational
journey / Alan Hobson & Cecilia Hobson.

ISBN 0-9685263-1-4

1. Hobson, Alan, 1958- --Health. 2. Hobson, Cecilia, 1957-.
3. Leukemia--Patients--Alberta--Biography. I. Hobson, Cecilia, 1957-
II. Title.

RC643.H62 2004   362.1'9699419'0092   C2003-906026-8

Printed and bound in Canada by Friesens, Altona, Manitoba, www.friesens.com
First Printing, October 2004.

ACKNOWLEDGMENTS

It is impossible to thank the thousands of people to whom Cecilia and I owe our lives and without whom this story would not have been possible. Notwithstanding, we would like to thank those mentioned in drafts of the book. For anyone we have inadvertently missed, we sincerely apologize and request your understanding.

Missy and Ken Allen

Steven Aung

Halina and Bolek Babiarz

Jo Ann and the late Rod Barnes

Debbie Baylin

Mike Bellos

Peter Beyak

Mike Bonnaventure

Marilyn Bouchard

Chris Brown

Linda Brown

Ahsan Chaudry

Jamie Clarke

John Clarke

Jim Cleghorn

Carol Davis

Shane Devlin

Rita, Brian, Garret and
  Breanne Dillabough

Rick Elliott

Cathy, Dale and Georgia Ens

Christian Fibich

Delia, Wilfred and the late
  Wayde Gallant

Niceto Gile

Graham Hawkes

Carl Hiebert

Jane, Daniel, Michael, Taryn and the
  late Peter James Hobson

Diane, Eric, Laura and
  Shannon Hobson

Isabel and the late Peter Hobson

Anne, James, Sarah and
  David Hobson

Derek Holt

Allan Jones

Laura Karlsson

Bruce Kirkby

Stephanie, Rae, Andrew,
  Stephen and Sarah Kopeechuk

Hal Kuntze

Terry Laughlin

Helen MacRae

Karen and the late Bill March

Patti and Natalee Mayer

Bill McDonald

John, Alicia and Leanne McIsaac

Bob and Brian McKenzie

Michael Menchel

James Nelson

Denny Netik

Kim Newhouse

Stephen Norris

Maurice O'Callaghan

Greg Ogilvie

Christine Pitkanen

Man-Chiu Poon

Peter Porcellato

Judy Ranson

Harry Rhoads, Jr.

Doug Rovira

Ben Ruether

Jim Russell

Karen Sabo

David Sadler

Valerie and Laura Simonson

Laurie Skreslet

David Smith

Delsie Sordi

Carol Spitzer

Jane Stewart

Bernie Swain

Mary Tidlund

the late Rob Tingley

Nomi Whalen

Tara Whittaker

Tracy Wuth (Amiss)

Cal Zaryski

We chose many people to help us with this highly personal and sensitive material. A very special thanks goes to Marie Lovgren, our business manager, who took on the Herculean task of contacting the over one hundred people mentioned in the over one dozen drafts of the book, liaised with other publishers, performed important editorial research and coordinated design and printing. If this book is a success, it is due in no small part to her professionalism, attention to detail and commitment to excellence.

We owe a special debt of gratitude to Janet Alford. Were it not for her collaboration, probing questions, patience and encouragement, Cecilia's voice might never have been heard. We would have been lost without her insight and support.

We are also indebted to the following individuals for their invaluable editorial and production contributions:

For manuscript review: Debbie Baylin, Mary Cook, Dale Ens, Jane and Dan Hobson, Gail and Bruce Leavens, Sylvia McAlister and Gareth Thomson, Sue and Bob McKenzie, Cheryl and Bob Nolda, and Anastasia Toufexis

For medical review: Dr. Chris Brown, Dr. Man-Chiu Poon and Dr. Jim Russell

For editing: Janet Alford, Martin Blumenauer, Leslie Johnson, Shauna Toh and Anastasia Toufexis

For front, back and inside dust jacket photography:
Brad Wrobleski and Michelle Gilbert, Cirque Dynamics, Cochrane, Alberta

For graphic design: Gary Hewitt, Wedge.a&d, Calgary, Alberta

For proofreading: Debbie Baylin, Martin Blumenauer, Mary Cook, Dale Ens, Jane Hobson, Marie Lovgren and Kathleen Wiebe

For research and liaison: Janet Boyd and Marie Lovgren

For photo production and coordination: Cindy Yaunish and Marie Lovgren

Grateful acknowledgment is made to the following publishers for permission to reprint previously published material:

G. P. Putnam's Sons, New York, for Lance Armstrong/Sally Jenkins' book, *It's Not About the Bike*, pp. 73-74, 2000.

Disney Publishing Worldwide Inc., New York, for Dr. Marty Becker and Danelle Morton's *The Healing Power of Pets*, published by Hyperion, New York, p. 80, 2002.

Putnam Publishing Group, New York, for Robert Service's book, *Collected Poems of Robert Service*, p. 168, reprint edition, 2003.

Trademarks appearing in this book are the property of their respective owners and are used only to identify them and/or their respective products and services. Any errors, omissions or oversights are unintended. We wish to thank the following organizations for the use of their trademarks:

Amgen Inc. for NEUPOGEN
Canadian Breast Cancer Foundation for Run for the Cure
Canadian Imperial Bank of Commerce for CIBC
Canfield, Mr. John T. and Hansen, Mr. Mark V. for Chicken Soup for the Soul
Colts & Old Port Cigar Company for Colts
DaimlerChrysler for Dodge Challenger
DC Comics for Superman
FasTrak Systems, Inc. for Camelbak
GlaxoSmithKline plc for Zofran and Wellbutrin
The Goodyear Tire & Rubber Company for Goodyear
Hershey Foods Corporation for Reese's Pieces
Kraft Foods Holdings, Inc. for JELL-O
Legacy Hotels Corporation for The Palliser
Mars, Inc. for M&M's
Novartis AG for Neoral
The Pillsbury Company for Doughboy
Polar Electro Oy for Polar
Python (Monty) Pictures Limited for Monty Python
Reckitt & Coleman (Overseas) Ltd., for Neet
Sanofi-Sythélabo Inc. for Demerol
S.C. Johnson Home Storage, Inc. for Ziploc
Sun Ice Ltd. for sun ice
Total Immersion Inc. for Total Immersion
Warner-Lambert Company for Benadryl

A HIGHER PURPOSE

"There is no height, no depth, that the spirit of man,
guided by a higher spirit, cannot attain."

– Sir John Hunt,
Leader,
1953 British Everest Expedition,
First Team to Climb Mt. Everest

A portion of the revenues from the sale of this book
is contributed to *The Climb Back from Cancer Foundation*
to help cancer patients, survivors and caregivers climb back to better lives.
For more information, see the postscript.

DEDICATION

To the cast of thousands who helped save a life and who made our dream of a life together possible, those precious souls we met and those we have yet to meet. We owe you a debt that can never be repaid and we are grateful beyond words.

You are all living human treasures.

TABLE OF CONTENTS

Chapters

TABLE OF CONTENTS
(continued)

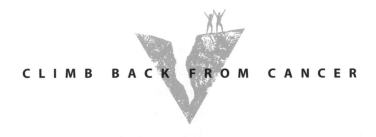

CLIMB BACK FROM CANCER

PREFACE

"Hope is our salvation from fear,
our strength amid struggle."

– Cecilia and Alan Hobson

Mahatma Gandhi once said: "Every worthwhile accomplishment, big or little, has its stages of drudgery and triumph; a beginning, a struggle and a victory."

The purpose of this book is to inspire you to achieve your own victory.

You may not be an Everest summiteer or the partner of one, but the skills that helped ensure our survival were not physical. They were psychological. They are not unique to us or to anyone. We all have these skills and capacities within us.

When it comes to cancer, the playing field is level. The disease does not discriminate based on marital status, gender, wealth, nationality, physical fitness or any of the other thousand and one variables we often use to define ourselves. We did not prepare for it anymore than you did. It just hit us like a semi-trailer. We did our best to survive the impact, get up and try to climb back.

You can too. When it comes to cancer, *anyone* can climb back – anyone.

That is why it does not matter if you have never climbed a mountain or anything higher than a flight of stairs. It does not even matter if you cannot climb stairs at all. This book is for anyone affected by cancer who wants to add quality to his or her life. It does not offer a guarantee of survival. It offers insight into how to maximize the chances of surviving, or at least living with dignity and courage in the time that is left. Despite what doctors may tell us, no one knows how long each of us has left.

Everyone has some kind of mountain to climb in life. At times, all of us are frightened; all of us can become overwhelmed. That is not only the essence of the cancer experience; it is the quintessence of life. But if we focus on our minds, our souls and on each other, and let our professional caregivers focus on our bodies, miracles can happen. One did for us. It may for you too.

Dr. Man-Chiu Poon, an oncologist you will meet in this book, puts it this way: "I put my fifty percent in and the patient puts his fifty percent in and together we have a chance. But if the patient doesn't put his half in, we only have half a chance."

We cannot afford to have half a chance when we are trying to climb "The Everest of Illnesses." We must have a whole chance and we must have a whole team – survivor, caregivers, family, friends, relatives, colleagues, associates – pulling together. Survivors cannot do it alone. The challenge is too big. But together we can make it to the top. Together we can triumph.

There is a mountain of strength that exists within us all at this moment, a treasure house we all have, but rarely explore. It is this psychological storehouse we must now tap into. If we do, we can unlock something inestimably powerful.

Without question, this has been an extremely difficult book to write. Cancer is a hard subject to write about, not only because it is a painful subject, but also because it can be painful to relive pain – repeatedly. Each of the over twelve drafts this manuscript has gone through released strong feelings in us. In that sense, this book has been both cathartic and harrowing to produce. It took us over three years to write. We persisted because we believe it will help others. We hope you are one of them.

In addition to this book, we hope that *"The Climb Back from Cancer Collection"* may eventually include *Climb Back from Cancer – Book II* and hopefully, *Book III* as well. In later books, we may explore the key psychological skills and how-to's we believe were central to our survival and success amid life-threatening illness. This book *(Book I)* concludes with a brief introduction to those skills. We call them *"The 10 Tools of Triumph"* for survivors and caregivers. There are ten skills for survivors and ten for caregivers – twenty in total. Each is highlighted once in the text. All twenty of the tools appear again in the conclusion. We believe these tools may help you in your current climb. We also close with a postscript that brings you up to date on what has happened in our lives since the final chapter, as well as a brief summary of what worked for us physically, psychologically and spiritually in our climb back. We leave you with a few sources for more information and a short list of some recommended reading. We hope all of this will give you enough inspiration and information to keep you climbing with greater conviction and courage.

So, here is our story. May you draw strength from it as we have drawn strength from those of others. Your struggle and ours is a shared one and potentially a shared victory – whether we define victory as a climb back to a new life or a climb up to another dimension. Regardless of the peak we seek to scale, we must hold fast to each other and to our dreams. Hope is our salvation from fear, our strength amid struggle. It is the path to the peak and the trail to victory.

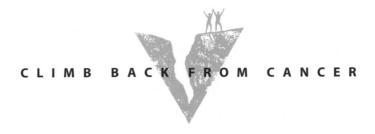

INTRODUCTION

"If we're persistent enough, we can do the dreams."

– Alan Hobson

On May 23, 1997, during my third expedition to Mount Everest, I finally stood on the top of the world. It was a pretty magnificent moment. I could see for what seemed like a hundred miles in all directions. It was a brilliant, blue-sky day. There was not a breath of wind. As I looked out over the world from my rarefied perch at 29,035 feet, I could actually see the horizon bending in my peripheral vision. Above me, I knew the atmosphere ultimately gave way to outer space and the limitless universe beyond. I felt simultaneously triumphant and infinitesimally small.

It took me thirty-nine years to see my childhood dream come true. It was a glorious and powerful fifteen minutes. "If we're persistent enough," I radioed down to base camp from the highest physical point on the planet, my voice cracking with emotion, "we can do the dreams." Tears of joy froze to my face.

After Everest I was at peace, if only temporarily. On a physical level at least, I no longer had to prove anything to anyone, especially myself. It was liberating. For a year, my goal was to not have a goal. All my life, whether as a student, gymnast, writer, journalist, speaker or adventurer, I had been a human *doing*. Now I wanted to be a human *being* – and just *be* from moment to moment.

This approach worked for a few months, but as I gradually recovered physically, psychologically and emotionally from the intense Everest experience, my ambition began to return. So did the same question over and over again from others: "So…what's next? How are you going to top Everest?" I quickly tired of hearing it and even began to resent it. To me, the question somehow reduced Everest to a thirty-second sound bite on the evening news, an achievement that was significant only if it was swiftly followed by something perceived as greater – perhaps a trip into outer space? But after that, then what – Mars, Jupiter or Pluto? At some point, the discussion became inane.

I have never really resolved the conflict between doing and being in my life. Much of the world does not seem to acknowledge people for just *being* anymore – except, of course, if they are being loving, as Mother Teresa was; compassionate, as the Dalai Lama is; or generous, as Bill Gates has been (after *doing* the incredible by building a global business empire). If we are *being* of service to others, that is a great thing, but the world mostly seems to recognize things we *do* – in my case, adventuring, writing books and making speeches. So, reaching the top of Everest created a peculiar personal dilemma for me. If I was no longer climbing the world's highest peak, what was I doing?

Someone once said: "If we are what we do, then when we don't do, we aren't." Thus, the very act of stepping to the top of the world sent me to the bottom of a self-identity crisis that seemed almost as deep as the mountain was high.

Three years after Everest, on August 10, 2000, I finally got the answer to the question "What's next?" and ultimately some insight into who I am as a human *being*. On that day, any illusions I might have had about my own immortality evaporated with three simple words: "You have cancer." That is when, at the age of forty-two, I was stripped of my previous identity. It was then that I started up a mountain higher, harder and more frightening than any I have ever climbed. That is when I learned I might have less than a year to live.

None of us knows how long we are going to live. As much as we would like to control how long we live, we cannot, because ultimately (and here is a big one), we are not in control. However, *how* we live is far more important than how long we live and that *is* something within our control.

My climb back from cancer was arduous and sometimes terrifying. Surprisingly, it was some of the life lessons I had learned on Everest and through other experiences that were so valuable to me in the climb. I have therefore included some of these lessons, excerpts from my previous books, in this book. We do not have to go to Everest to apply them.

The climbing plan on my medical mountain included around-the-clock, high dose chemotherapy and an adult blood stem cell transplant – one of the most radical and risky medical procedures known. If I had faced this kind of a challenge on my own, I would never have survived. Fortunately, I had "Sherpas" with me.

The Sherpas are the mountain people of Nepal. They are neither porters nor guides. They have evolved into the strongest high altitude climbers in the world – bar none. More Sherpas have been to the summit of Everest than any other nationality or cultural group. Because they are born and live at 13,000 feet and above, they have a 13,000-foot acclimatization advantage over those of us who live at sea level or thereabouts. They are colossally strong, capable of carrying loads of up to one hundred and fifty pounds (about the weight of the average household refrigerator) at elevations as extreme as 22,000 feet and incredibly, sometimes higher.

But it is not their physical strength that makes them so special. It is their spiritual strength. They refer to Everest as "Chomolungma," the Tibetan word that means "Mother Goddess of the World." As devout Buddhists, the Sherpas are meek, gentle and humble. They never complain. There are only two things fierce about them – their courage and their loyalty. There have been numerous instances in which Sherpas have lost their fingers and toes to frostbite trying to rescue Westerners in the Himalayas. Many have even lost their lives. They believe that when you set foot in the world's tallest mountain range, you have entered their home and, therefore, your safety is one hundred percent their responsibility. In general, the Sherpas have received little credit for the thousands of Everest expeditions in which they have participated.

As I wrote in my previous book, *From Everest to Enlightenment*:

> *I believe we are all Sherpas carrying loads of one sort or another. And we find ourselves struggling up our own mountains – whether they are professional, personal, marital, emotional, interpersonal, parental, medical or financial. At times, some of us cannot seem to find the strength to bear our burdens. The path we're on seems brutally steep and unrelenting. Sometimes [as TV anchorman Howard Beale in the 1976 movie classic, Network, said], "We just can't take it any more." We sit exhausted and disillusioned by the side of the trail and hope that somehow the crushing weight on our shoulders will magically be lifted or at least lightened. Our hearts are heavy, as are our souls.*
>
> *Whatever path we have chosen in life, climb we must, for to do otherwise is to relinquish our own self-respect and give in to our frailties and fear.*

On my medical mountain, I had the benefit of many "Sherpa caregivers." They did not come from Nepal, but they had the same attributes as their Eastern equivalents. They were incredibly strong-willed, courageous and loyal. Their contributions were absolutely vital and largely unrecognized.

I believe that the presence of Sherpa caregivers in the life of a cancer patient substantially increases that patient's odds of survival, or at the very least, the quality of life for the time left. These Sherpas do not only carry physical loads. They help carry the emotional, social, financial, logistical and parental burdens cancer treatment inevitably creates. Yet most of the attention and care goes to the patient. Because of this, the weight Sherpa caregivers must carry is often heavier than that of the patient. It is the patient who is facing the prospect of potential death, but it is the caregivers who, in addition to managing their own lives and fears, must help manage the patient's as well.

In the Himalayas, this is called "carrying a double load." It means that instead of shouldering a fifty-pound pack – a substantial weight even at sea level, a Nepalese Sherpa must carry a hundred pounds or more. Sherpa caregivers must also shoulder their burdens in a life-threatening situation. While the patient is struggling to climb back, the Sherpa caregivers are shoulder-to-shoulder with them, carrying two metaphorical sleeping bags, two tents, two stoves, and twice the food, fuel and oxygen along the terrifying exposed ridges and across the hazardous avalanche slopes. Theirs is a very heavy pack and their path is treacherous.

In my climb back, I was truly blessed with the presence of many Sherpa caregivers – individuals who saw my plight, tied into my rope and climbed with me. One such Sherpa was my then fiancée, Cecilia. Two years after my diagnosis, I knew her and she knew me more intimately than some couples who have been married for fifty years. My story is her story. In fact, it is our story because as you will see, I would not be alive were it not for Cecilia.

The ultimate goal of a Sherpa is to pass into the next life having made the lives of as many others around them as rich as possible. The virtue to which they most aspire is not financial wealth, material possessions, position, power or fame. It is compassion for all living things

– From Everest to Enlightenment

You may not have a Cecilia Sherpa or a background in high altitude mountaineering. There may be no known medical "cure" for your disease, or the prognosis may be bleak. Regardless of the circumstances, if we are to survive a medical mountain as challenging as cancer, or at least live out the rest of the time we have left with as much quality of life as possible, we must seek out Sherpa caregivers immediately. They can be doctors, nurses, personal care assistants, associates, friends or family members – in fact, anyone with whom we come in contact. We must have the courage to ask them to share our load because in a hospital or hospice, just as in the Himalayas, there is strength in numbers.

Dr. Greg Ogilvie, Director of the Animal Cancer Center at the Colorado State University College of Veterinary Medicine in Fort Collins, Colorado, wrote: "Cancer represents the summit of the lack of hope." Regardless of how we see it, if we believe life-threatening illness is a death sentence, we are dead. But if we think of it as a "life sentence" call to action, there is hope.

This is the story of our climb back from cancer. As any cancer patient knows, that climb does not have a summit. It will never end until our lives do. Either the presence of cancer or the fear of it will always be with us. We do not just heal and get better after cancer like healing after a broken bone. We heal and then, if we are lucky, we get on with our lives as best we can for whatever time we have, in whatever way we can, with whatever faculties we have. The prospect of a relapse or metastasis never goes away. It is always there, sometimes as a distant anxiety, sometimes as a big black thunderhead parked directly overhead.

For every mountain we climb in life, another appears before us more daunting than the one before. So come with us now as we climb this "Inner Everest." It is a world of hostile weather, thin air and an elusive summit. Yet this book is not about *doing* anything except rising to a challenge. It is about *being* – being tested, being tenacious and being triumphant. Our dream is to give you or someone you know the most powerful climbing tool of all – hope.

CAST OF CHARACTERS

Some of the Thousands Who Helped Save a Life
and Who Made a New Life for Us Together Possible

(in alphabetical order, see photographs that follow)

Ken Allen
Alan's university gymnastics coach

Bolek Babiarz
one of Alan's personal care assistants in hospital

Rod and Jo Ann Barnes
one of Alan's fellow patients and his wife/caregiver

Jim Cleghorn
one of Alan's fellow patients

Rita Dillabough
one of Alan's acute care nurses

Dale, Cathy and Georgia Ens
Alan's best friend, his wife and their daughter

Dr. Christian Fibich
one of Alan's outpatient oncologists

Daniel, Jane, Michael and Taryn Hobson
Alan's eldest brother, sister-in-law, nephew and niece.
Michael had a bone marrow transplant in 1994.

Eric Hobson
Alan's second eldest brother. Alan's adult blood stem cell donor.

Isabel and Peter Hobson
Alan's parents

James Hobson
Alan's twin brother

Andrew, Stephanie, Rae, Stephen and Sarah Kopeechuk
one of Alan's fellow patients, Andrew's mother, father, adult blood stem cell
donor brother, and sister

Dr. Helen MacRae
Alan and Cecilia's psychologist

Patti Mayer
Alan's friend, physiotherapist, acupuncturist and Reiki practitioner

Bob McKenzie
Alan and Eric's cousin and friend. Eric's business partner.

Dr. Man-Chiu Poon
one of Alan's hematologists

Harry Rhoads, Jr.
President of the Washington Speakers Bureau

Dr. Jim Russell
Alan's adult blood stem cell transplant oncologist

Valerie Simonson
Alan's meditation instructor and friend

Laurie Skreslet
Alan's friend and mentor, the first Canadian to climb Mt. Everest

Bernie Swain
CEO of the Washington Speakers Bureau

Cal Zaryski
one of Alan's exercise physiologists, his personal
training coach and friend

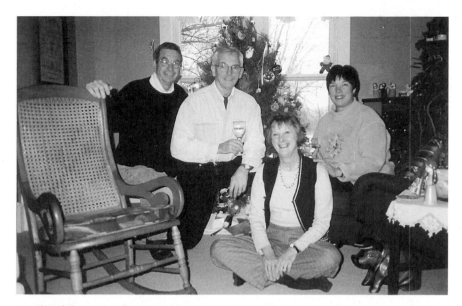

1. A Pivotal Figure: Alan's former university gymnastics coach, Ken Allen (second from left), is flanked by Gary Coll, one of Alan's former journalism professors; Elaine Coll (second from right) and Missy Allen.

Alan: *"Ken has been one of the greatest influences in my life. The lessons I learned in his gym paid off handsomely in my cancer journey. 'Our attitude at the beginning of a task largely determines our attitude at the end of a task,' he once told me."*

Photo Credit: Ken Allen

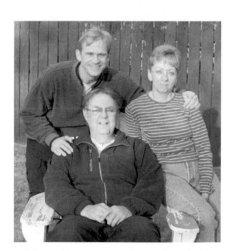

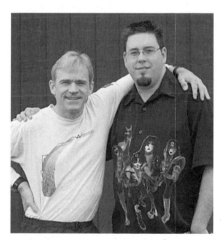

2. A Potent Force: Alan (standing) with Rod and Jo Ann Barnes.

Alan: *"Cecilia and I agreed that if we could muster a fraction of Rod and Jo Ann's resolve, perhaps the four of us would one day meet again outside the ward. They showed us that although mountaineers could be tough, a night warehouseman and his wife could be tougher."*

Photo Credit: Cecilia Hobson

3. A Fighter: Alan with fellow leukemia survivor, Jim Cleghorn.

Alan: *"Like me, Jim hated the confinement of the hospital and wanted nothing more than to escape it as soon as possible. Unlike me, he fought every step of the way. He wanted to live to have his own car audio business."*

Photo Credit: Cecilia Hobson

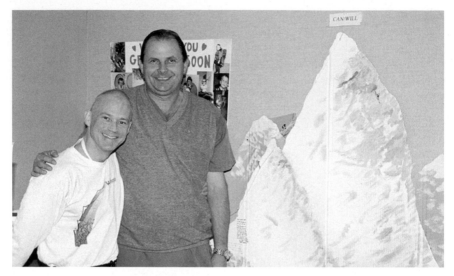

4. The Medical Mountain: Alan with personal care assistant Bolek Babiarz and his amazing creation.

Alan: *"It was a cardboard cutout he had made of three 'mountains.' On one end was Mt. Everest, on the other was its sister peak, Mt. Lhotse, and in the middle, the biggest of the three peaks, was my medical mountain. A little handwritten note along the bottom read: 'Consider this another mountain to climb in your life, Alan, so be strong. Never give up my friend.'"*

Photo Credit: Cecilia Hobson

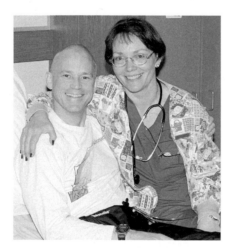

5. The Answer to a Prayer: Alan with acute care nurse, Rita Dillabough.

Alan: *"Her touch was light and soothing, and she moved as effortlessly around the hospital room as she would around her own living room. Her glasses encircled eyes that twinkled brightly, and they instantly communicated compassion and care. From the moment we met her, Cecilia and I knew she had been divinely sent."*

Photo Credit: ABL Imaging

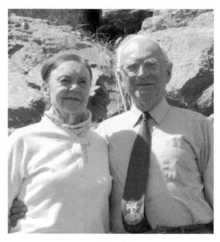

6. Founding Forces: Alan's parents, Isabel and Peter Hobson.

Alan: *"How do you tell your parents that a child they love might predecease them? Given my parents' previous cancer experience with my two nephews, I feared they might take my cancer diagnosis hard."*

Photo Credit: Alan Hobson

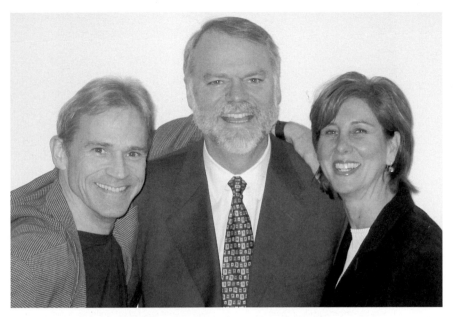

7. A Bona Fide Hero: Alan and Cecilia enjoy a lighter moment with Alan's brother and adult blood stem cell donor, Eric.

Cecilia: *"Eric's personality is much different than Alan's. Eric is constantly joking and his laugh is contagious. Although he's an ambitious businessman, he knows how to relax and have fun. Perhaps Alan will acquire some of Eric's lightheartedness through the transplant. I can only hope."*

Photo Credit: Bruce Hobson

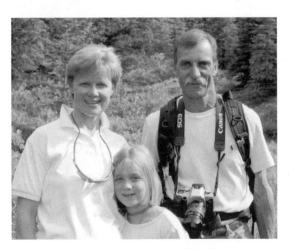

8. Equanimity in Action: Our close friends, Cathy, Georgia and Dale Ens.

Alan: *"Dale explained that with my power of attorney, he and Cecilia would take care of my business, bills, will, medical directives and all my financial affairs. 'You only need to concentrate on one thing,' he counseled, '– getting better. For the next six months, that's where I want you to put your entire focus. We'll take care of the rest.'"*

Photo Credit: Alan Hobson

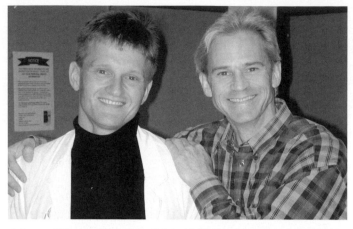

9. Creator of History: Alan with Dr. Christian Fibich, his outpatient oncologist.

Alan: *"Cancer survivors are often plagued by chronic fatigue. When my exhaustion vanished as a result of mild aerobic activity, Dr. Fibich quickly wrote the protocol for a medical study. One cancer survivor who had only been able to work part-time on and off in the eight years following a bone marrow transplant because of chronic fatigue went back to work full-time within one month of beginning the physical activity program that was part of the study."*

Photo Credit: Cecilia Hobson

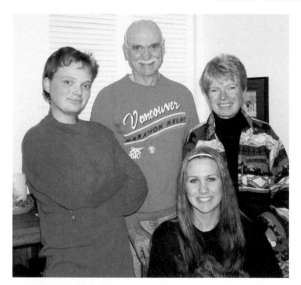

10. Living Courage: Alan's brother, Daniel Hobson, with his wife, Jane, and their children, Michael and Taryn.

Alan: *"Dan and Jane lost their first-born son, Peter James, to leukemia thirteen years earlier. Their second son, Michael, came down with a similar condition a few years later and had a successful bone marrow transplant. Somehow, through all this, Dan had kept his job, his health and his marriage to Jane intact. They had gone on to adopt a wonderful little girl, Taryn, and they had raised her and Michael with a conviction that loss could be overcome by love."*

Photo Credit: Heather Van Tassel

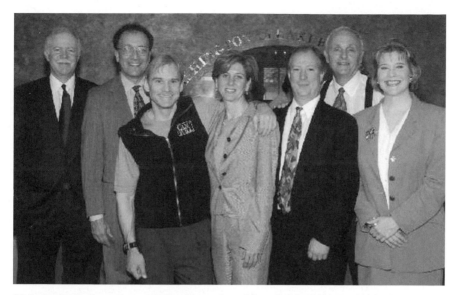

11. An Impressive Team: Alan and Cecilia with members of the staff of the Washington Speakers Bureau, (L-R) President Harry Rhoads, Jr., Vice President Michael Menchel, Vice President Bob Parsons, CEO Bernie Swain and Event Coordinator Malinda Waughtal.

Alan: *"When the bureau's two founding partners learned of my diagnosis, they immediately asked when I wanted them to fly out to see me. 'You will survive this,' they said insistently, 'and when you do, you will be an even better presenter because of it. Just let us know when you're ready to speak again. We'll block off the calendar for as long as you need.'"*

Photo Credit: Washington Speakers Bureau

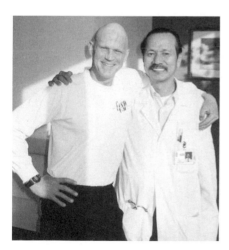

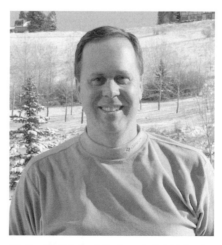

12. The First Man In: Alan with hematologist, Dr. Man-Chiu Poon, who made Alan's initial diagnosis of acute leukemia.

Alan: *"With his shoot-from-the-hip, no-holds-barred bedside manner, Dr. Poon earned my instant respect as a physician who had the guts to tell it like it was."*

Photo Credit: J.P. Hobson

13. Good Folk Indeed: Alan's cousin, Bob McKenzie.

"'My grandmother once told me that good folk are few,' Bob said. 'When you find them, keep them, nurture them. They are precious.'"

Photo Credit: Spring Webb

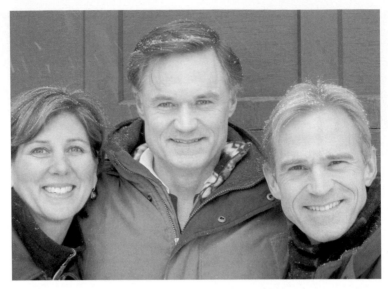

14. The Brinkman: Cecilia and Alan with Alan's twin brother, James.

Alan: *"James made his living as a computer consultant and was responsible for helping maintain the software that tracked the Prime Minister's correspondence from the public and generated swift replies. It was a task that required around-the-clock vigilance, a methodical mind and above all, a cool head. My father called James a 'brinkman.' He was good at the edge."*

Photo Credit: Daniel Hobson

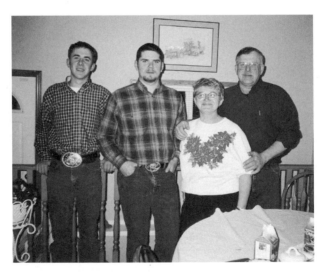

15. The Strength of a Bull: Alan's fellow leukemia survivor, Andrew Kopeechuk (second from left), with his brother, Stephen, who donated his adult blood stem cells to Andrew, and their parents, Stephanie and Rae Kopeechuk.

Alan: *"I knew immediately that Andrew's mind was in the right place because hanging from the television set in his hospital room, written in his own hand, were the words: 'I will get through this.'"*

Photo Credit: Sarah Kopeechuk (Andrew's sister)

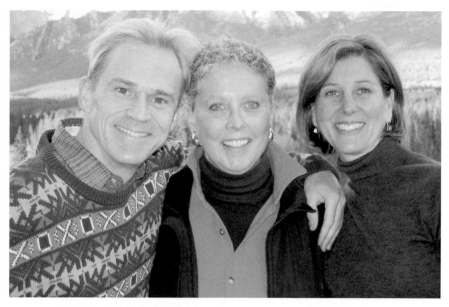

16. "Sage" Helen: Our psychologist, Dr. Helen MacRae.

"'This experience will take you to a place you have never been to before in your lives,' Helen said. 'Depending on how you both handle it, you will either grow together as a couple or you will grow apart. The enemy is not cancer. The enemy is fear.'"

Photo Credit: Dianne Roulson

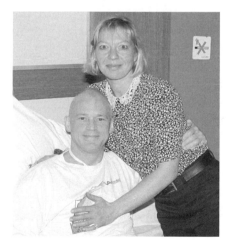

17. Sunshine on Legs: Alan with his friend, physiotherapist, acupuncturist and Reiki practitioner, Patti Mayer.

Alan: *"Patti never went anywhere at half speed. She was energetic and vital and she moved with a spring in her step and a mission in her heart. She wanted to positively affect every person with whom she came in contact."*

Photo Credit: ABL Imaging

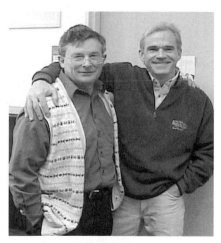

18. A Quiet Giant: Alan with Dr. Jim Russell, his transplant oncologist.

Alan: *"Jim may have been an elite doctor, but he was not an elitist. He never introduced himself as 'Dr. Russell,' only Jim. He was unpretentious, quiet and perceptive, always sensitive to the needs of others. Cecilia and I called him 'Gentle Jim.'"*

Photo Credit: Cecilia Hobson

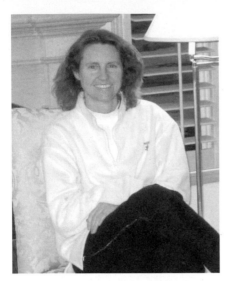

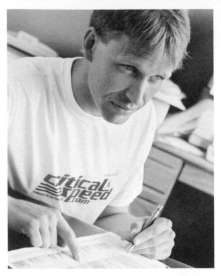

19. A Spiritual Sister: Our friend and Raja Yoga meditation instructor, Valerie Simonson.

Cecilia: *"Valerie is another healer who blesses us. When I return home at night and nestle into bed, I reach for my sleeping aid, a meditation tape. During those nights when I listen to the tape, my dreams are comforting and I awake feeling rested."*

Photo Credit: Valerie Simonson

20. Coach Cal: Cal Zaryski, Alan's personal training coach and friend, tracking the results of physical activity. Cal helped oversee Alan's climb back from cancer and now helps other cancer survivors do the same, in person and on-line.

Alan: *"While I pedaled the bike, Cal looked on as I was hooked up to a machine that analyzed the gases expelled in my breath. Soon Dr. Smith declared: 'Congratulations. You are remarkably fit for a guy who has been through a near-death experience, but we detect from your results that you have been exercising too hard. Try reducing your intensity and you may see improvements.' It worked. Within weeks, I noticed an increase in my energy to a level that approached that of pre-transplant. If this worked for me, would it work for others?"*

Photo Credit: Darren Zaryski

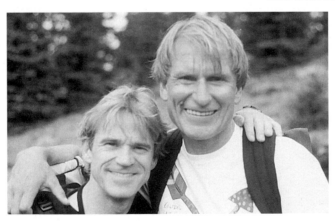

21. A Mentor: Alan with his look-alike friend and fellow speaker, Laurie Skreslet, the first Canadian to climb Mt. Everest.

Alan: *"When Laurie finished talking, he wrapped me once again in his arms and whispered something in my ear I will never forget: 'When we run away from fear, it gets bigger,' he stated with conviction, 'but when we advance towards it, it shrinks.'"*

Photo Credit: Dale Ens

CHAPTER 1

Alan

A NEW MOUNTAIN BECKONS

The mountain gave me what I needed and it wasn't just the summit. It was a positive sense of closure with Everest and the deep satisfaction of knowing that I had given it everything I had, short of my life. I had fulfilled my mission. The summit was a bonus. Now I could finish a chapter in my life and begin a new one.

– From Everest to Enlightenment

It had been an unsettling couple of weeks. What began as a routine visit to my family doctor had rapidly escalated into something more.

I made the initial appointment because I had been plagued for months by a persistent sore throat, swollen glands and fatigue. The doctor diagnosed a harmless case of post-nasal drip and prescribed antibiotics. But a week later, things had not improved and I went back. This time I insisted on a blood test. It revealed that the hemoglobin in my blood, the part that transports oxygen, was unusually low. My physician urged me to see a specialist immediately. Unfortunately, that specialist would not be able to see me at his office. I would have to go to the local cancer center.

That is when I first heard the dreaded "C" word in association with my health. In the past, whenever I had driven past the Tom Baker Cancer Centre, I had thanked my lucky stars I was not in there. Terrible things happened there, I imagined. I did not want to go *there*!

My family doctor would not allow my anxiety to overcome my need. On the insistence of one of the nurses in her office, I showed up for my rush appointment with the hematologist the next day, accompanied by my fiancée, Cecilia.

At the cancer center, after a quick visit to the blood lab where I gave another sample, Cecilia and I took a seat in the waiting room of the day clinic. There, a nurse handed me a questionnaire.

"What have you been told about the type of cancer you have?" one question asked.

I bristled.

"No one has told me I have cancer," I wrote, wondering what the hell was going on. I had just given a blood sample minutes before.

"What kind of a question is that?" I asked Cecilia as she sat next to me. "These guys should be a little bit more sensitive to the fact that not *everyone* who comes in here has cancer. Obviously there's been some kind of a mix-up."

Twenty minutes passed. Anxiously, we waited for my name to be called.

The next eyes we looked into were Dr. Poon's. They telegraphed intensity. He stood before us in a long white lab coat, the collar of a blue dress shirt and white undershirt visible beneath it. His thin black hair was combed straight back behind his high forehead and he spoke in a hoarse low voice thick with a Chinese accent. It demanded attention. He was about my height, five foot six, but despite a light frame and fine features, he projected the aura of a man twice his size. With a deeply furrowed brow, he took one look at the results of my blood test and probed: "So tell me, how have you been feeling?"

"Not too good," I said. "Too tired."

"I see," he replied forebodingly.

Then he said he wanted to take a biopsy. That is when things got really scary.

Bone marrow biopsies sound bad – and I mean literally *sound*. Cecilia held my hand while Dr. Poon twisted the six-inch-long needle into my hip like he was screwing into hardwood. I could hear him puffing. Cecilia saw him sweating. Fortunately, I did not feel any pain thanks to a local anesthetic, but it was still alarming to have someone digging into me with a sharp instrument. I was not sure how to react, so I just looked at the blank white wall ahead of me and talked to a Higher Power.

The preliminary results of the biopsy suggested what Dr. Poon had suspected the minute he had looked at the results of my blood test. This was not any garden-variety low-grade infection. My situation could be serious.

The next day he called us at home.

"I thought you had chronic leukemia," the hoarse voice ventured, "but actually, I think you have acute leukemia."

"Acute?" I said. "What do you mean?"

"I mean you may not have a lot of time," he cautioned, "but I'll know more next week after we do further tests on your marrow sample. By then, I should have a more definitive diagnosis."

"Oh," I said, struggling to understand.

"I'll let you know then," he said.

Shell-shocked, I hung up. For a long time, I could not speak.

"What is it?" Cecilia pressed. "I heard you say 'acute.' Acute what?"

"Leukemia," I said.

She gasped.

"He's not yet sure, my love," I wrestled out the words, "so we shouldn't jump to conclusions, but it sounds like he's pretty sure."

"Pretty sure of what?" she probed.

"Pretty sure it could be serious."

There was another long silence.

The magnitude of what was happening hit us like a semi-trailer, shattering our comfortable existence into shards. We had to get away. We had to walk and talk and think and do whatever we could to prepare for what lay ahead, even if it was the worst. We needed time away from this nightmare.

We had a favorite little cabin by a river in the mountains of southern Alberta. We went there for a few days. It was a three-hour drive and all the way I could not stop worrying whether Cecilia would stick around for the conclusion of this drama. I could not blame her if she did not. We were to be married in four months. By then, if Dr. Poon was right, I might be dead.

Somehow, she knew what I was thinking. When we got to the cabin, she handed me a little card.

"I am tied into your rope," it said in her handwriting. "We will climb this mountain together."

> *"I am tied into your rope.*
> *We will climb this mountain together."*
>
> – Cecilia Hobson

This was the first in what would be an endless cord of commitments Cecilia would make to me in the coming months. They were not the flashy displays of courage you see at the movies or on television. They were much deeper and more meaningful. This was love – quiet, solid, unshakable – the stuff of dreams, the stuff you only come across once in a lifetime if you are lucky and I had stumbled upon a mother lode. In its simplicity and purity, it went far beyond romance. It was absolute and powerful. It reminded me of the words of the American mountaineer, author and high altitude researcher, Charles Houston: "When men climb on a great mountain together, the rope between them is more than a mere physical aid to the ascent; it is a symbol of the spirit of the enterprise. It is a symbol of men banded together in a common effort of will and strength against their only true enemies: inertia, cowardice, greed, ignorance and all weaknesses of the spirit."

There could not have been a better way for Cecilia to tell me where she stood. She stood with me. Amid the fear, trauma and the unknown, we were together.

"What about the wedding?" I asked as I hugged her, my eyes welling with tears.

"We'll get married when you're better," she said confidently. "I'm not going anywhere."

The next day I tried to go for a jog but was once again reminded that I was going downhill fast. I looked up at the massive rock formations on which I had so clearly defined myself to that point in my life and I wondered if I would live to touch them again. They were sheer, jagged and exposed – the way I felt. If Dr. Poon's preliminary diagnosis proved true, I would find myself teetering on the edge. If he was wrong...well, that was unlikely. It was possible, but improbable.

The nights before our next appointment passed interminably, the days not much faster. Finally, we were face to face again with Dr. Poon.

"I confirm a diagnosis of acute myeloid leukemia," he said assuredly. "Without treatment, your prognosis is less than a year."

The words seemed to hang in the air of the examining room like sinister vapors twisting weightlessly. They hardly registered in my brain. They simply hung, like a noose.

I looked over at Cecilia to see how she was taking the news. Incredibly, she was taking notes.

My mind shot out one question. I knew cancer treatment often involved intensive chemotherapy. That scared me. So I asked Dr. Poon, "What if I do nothing?"

His answer sticks with me to this day: "You're screwed."

Startled by the directness of the reply, I asked him what treatment options I had. He explained that with chemotherapy, the chances of putting the leukemia into remission were about seventy percent. The problem was remission could be only temporary. If we were able to put my cancer into remission and if a possible donor match could be found fast enough, I might be able to receive a bone marrow or adult blood stem cell transplant that might "cure" me of the disease. Still, that was a lot of "ifs."

"So," he asked, "is the cup half empty or is it half full, Alan? The choice is yours."

"Is the cup half empty or is it half full?
The choice is yours."

– Dr. Man-Chiu Poon,
Hematologist

Dr. Man-Chiu Poon, a kind and internationally respected blood specialist with decades of experience treating cancer, was not being insensitive by bluntly telling me how serious my situation was. On the contrary, he had quickly decided how best to communicate with a strong-willed patient and he had read me perfectly. He had chosen to be brutally honest – and for good reason.

Acute leukemia is cancer of the blood. It is a potentially lethal condition during which there is a rapid and uncontrolled release of trillions of immature and ineffective white blood cells called "blasts" from the bone marrow into the blood stream. These blasts pour into the blood, quickly pushing aside all the healthy white blood cells used to combat disease, the red blood cells used to transport oxygen to the tissues and the platelets used to stop bleeding. A patient with acute leukemia can rapidly hemorrhage because of a low platelet count, die from infection due to ineffective white blood cells or get progressively weaker and weaker from anemia because of an insufficient number of oxygen-carrying red blood cells. Eighty-five percent of those diagnosed with the condition are dead within three years. Untreated, the disease is one hundred percent fatal. You cannot cut leukemia out with surgery or burn it out with radiation. Once the cancer is in your blood, it is in your whole body. Each year about 35,000 – about one in 10,000 North Americans – are diagnosed with the disease. Now, I was one of them.

Dr. Poon's biopsy of my bone marrow had shown that a frightening ninety percent of the cells in my bone marrow, the main manufacturing plant for blood cells, and forty percent of the cells in my bloodstream, were blasts. If the number of blasts in my bloodstream increased much more, or if I hemorrhaged or developed an infection, it was over for me. Dr. Poon knew he had to get my attention. With his shoot-from-the-hip, no-holds-barred bedside manner, he earned my instant respect as a physician who had the guts to tell it like it was.

"We need to admit you and begin intensive, around-the-clock chemotherapy right away," he said, his intense stare burning the severity of the situation into my stunned psyche. "Treatment will take at least four months. Would you like to begin Saturday?"

It was Thursday. With all due appreciation for Dr. Poon's lightning-swift attention to my case, this was still happening too fast. Given more time, I might be able to get my mind around the fact I had cancer, but double-barreled chemotherapy of the magnitude he was talking about was another leap altogether, to say nothing of shutting down my business and my life for at least four months. Our time away in the mountains had helped us to consider our options, but nothing could have prepared us for this moment. I was overwhelmed.

I could not accept that I had cancer of the blood. I did not want to lose my hair or the contents of my stomach repeatedly. I did not want to start popping pills like corner-store candy, experience endless blood transfusions or endure innumerable invasive bone marrow biopsies. I did not want to lose my savings, my vocation or my self-identity. I did not want to lose control, or what I perceived as control, of my whole life as I had known it. Mostly, I did not want to die; I wanted to live.

At moments like this, moments when the core of who we are is tested, we can either accept reality and the opinions of others or we can choose to reject them. That choice tests our character like no other experience in life.

In the past, I had faced other daunting choices. I had chosen to go back to Mt. Everest three times despite judgments that my first two expeditions had "failed." During both these attempts, although we had been unable to reach the summit, we had not failed to learn from our experiences. Our first expedition had missed the summit by 3,000 vertical feet, our second by just two city blocks. Ultimately, we had been able to take our first two attempts and turn them into a resounding triumph on our third trip.

It took me ten years of climbing and fundraising, ten expeditions to high altitude and decades of preparation to achieve my Everest dream. As far as I could see, a diagnosis of cancer was no different. Cancer was "The Everest of Illnesses." I was not going to get to the top of this mountain overnight either. If I hoped just to get out of base camp and survive the first few steps, I would have to get my head together quickly, think rationally and act as decisively as I could.

I could either choose to see my prognosis as an inevitable death sentence, as a failure to live beyond age forty-two, or as an opportunity to choose life, climb on and hope for the best. Most importantly, I first had to stop my mind from wildly spinning off into the future, extrapolating to catastrophe. I had to cancel the catastrophe – now – and stay one hundred percent present in the moment. For the moment, although my life was threatened, I was not in any imminent danger. There were no tigers lunging at me or roofs caving in from above. Emotionally, though, I felt like my world had imploded.

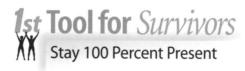

1st Tool for *Survivors*
Stay 100 Percent Present

The realization that my life might soon end did not come easily. I had spent forty-two years going after my dreams. Fear of critical illness had never really entered my mind until my five-year-old nephew, Peter James, had died of leukemia thirteen years earlier. A few years later, his younger brother, Michael, had developed a similar condition. Miraculously, Michael had received a successful bone marrow transplant from a man who worked for a sponsor of one of my Everest expeditions. Aside from that part of my family history, there was no sign whatsoever of critical illness in me or my family – no heart disease, diabetes, stroke or high blood pressure.

I remember as a boy having this strange feeling about how long I would live. For some reason, I could never seem to imagine anything beyond age forty-two. It was like there was a brick wall in my future.

In the three years since summiting Everest at age thirty-nine, I had worked incredibly hard at my speaking career – living on planes and in hotels all over North America and Europe, changing time zones, continents, countries and cities, missing meals, sacrificing sleep and pushing myself hard.

In theory, I lived in a two-bedroom apartment in Calgary, Alberta, Canada, just east of the Canadian Rocky Mountains. In reality, I lived on the road. I would fly in late at night, having traveled up to eighteen hours, get four or five hours of fitful sleep, make a presentation before hundreds or thousands of people early the next morning and fly out that afternoon to my next speaking engagement.

Extensive business travel with insufficient rest between trips is hard on the body and mind. The constant packing and unpacking, checking in and out of hotels, changing cities, airports and taxis, making flights, meeting with clients, exercising daily and performing at my peak on stage – all created an ongoing and unsettling anxiety. I was always running somewhere.

The American humorist, James Thurber, once wrote: "All men should try and learn before they die, what they are running from and to and why." I had been running from one speaking engagement to the next. Why? Because that is what I thought busy speakers were supposed to do. They were supposed to be busy. Perhaps I had become mentally, physically and emotionally burned out and my immune system had simply collapsed.

My personal adventures had also stressed my body and mind. High altitude climbing involves long periods of extreme exertion in low oxygen environments. This is accompanied by severe dehydration, prolonged exposure to intense ultraviolet rays and less-than-sanitary living conditions. Climbers sleep little and rest even less. After summiting Everest,

I remember my colleague, Jamie Clarke, remarking that he felt like his bone marrow was tired. That statement now shook me to my core. Maybe I had traveled, trained, fundraised, climbed, spoken and flown too far for too long. Perhaps these were the roots of my "dis-ease."

Needing to learn more about what might have caused my leukemia, I called Dr. Doug Rovira, a physician in Boulder, Colorado, who had been our expedition doctor during my last trip to Everest. Incredibly, he was an oncologist who specialized in leukemia, and his mother had died of the disease. He assured me firmly that there was no known link between a fast-paced lifestyle and leukemia. He said patients often added this kind of self-blame to their already considerable burden at the moment of diagnosis or later. They did this, he said, because they wished to feel like they could somehow pinpoint the cause of their condition so they might be able to control it, or if they survived, prevent it from recurring.

"Don't put that load of personal responsibility on your shoulders," Doug advised me forcefully. "You have more important things to think about than how and why this happened – like how you're going to get through it."

Nevertheless, my mind kept right on spinning. If Doug was right, my physical past had nothing to do with the onset of my illness. Then what about my emotional past?

Early in the post-Everest period of my life, my business partnership and friendship with fellow adventurer, Jamie Clarke, had come apart. We had spent probably the most intense decade of our lives organizing our involvement in three $1 million Everest expeditions, two of which we had financed, organized and climbed on ourselves. We had set out on this Everest odyssey with no money, no office, no staff and no experience in high altitude climbing. Amazingly, ten years later, we had stood triumphant on the top of Everest just two hours apart. But only a few months after our return to North America, our relationship had ended. The accumulated stress of organizing and participating in each expedition had progressively eroded our friendship and pushed it to the breaking point. In addition, neither one of us had been able to get past our intensely competitive natures. In hindsight, I believe that instead of recognizing each other's complementary strengths, we had competed for everything from speaking time on stage to editorial space in our books and films. This sad conclusion stood in stark contrast with our collective triumphs. Jamie went on to cross the world's largest sand desert, The Empty Quarter of Saudi Arabia, with his brother, Leigh, and one of our fellow adventurers, Bruce Kirkby. It was only the second time in history it had been done.

At the same time as my relationship with Jamie was coming apart, so was my engagement to a wonderful woman. A single mother of three children, she lived in a city on the prairies hundreds of miles from Calgary and worked as an elementary school teacher. Despite the distance that separated us, we had maintained a passionate long-distance relationship and had trekked together to Everest base camp prior to my eventual ascent. But when I returned from the mountain, just as had happened with Jamie, we could not seem to bring our two worlds back together. I could not bring myself to move away from my beloved Rocky Mountains, and I believe she could not see uprooting her children from friends, family and school to join me, an often absent and high-strung road warrior.

These two crushing personal losses, along with the sudden and deep depression I experienced after summiting Everest (because when you achieve a goal, you also lose it), had left me emotionally deflated. Like Jamie, I had gone looking for a new goal after Everest. I had found a brilliant ocean engineer in San Francisco who had the expertise, but not the capital, to build the world's first underwater craft to "fly" to the deepest point in the ocean – 36,000 feet down. He had the ability to open up the last physical frontier on the planet in much the same way the Wright brothers had opened up the skies. If I were able to raise the capital for what was called "The Ocean Everest Expedition," I might be able to help write a new chapter in world exploration and perhaps even become the first person to visit the highest and lowest points on the planet. Here was something exciting! Here was a way to fuel my passion for adventure.

The challenge was the staggering US $12 million needed to stage such an expedition. Confident I could raise the capital from my Fortune 500 corporate speaking clients, I committed to finding the money.

A few months into the project, I began to notice significant changes in my body. I could not swim more than a few lengths of the pool without becoming exhausted. At the same time, because I wear a heart rate monitor during physical activity, I noticed my pulse was unusually high. I had begun to feel run-down and lethargic. When I was not able to get through the day without taking a one- or two-hour nap in the afternoon, I knew something was seriously wrong. I had energy somewhere, but I just could not seem to connect to it.

These symptoms had persisted for a few months, but I had put them off as accumulated fatigue caused by speaking, traveling and fundraising for Ocean Everest. Then my Ocean Everest dream evaporated. I was not able to raise the money fast enough and my relationship with the project ended. It was another bitter disappointment in my attempt to re-define myself after Everest and my life began to look bleak.

As disappointing as the loss of Ocean Everest had been, however, my past had hardly been depressing. Two years before our meeting with Dr. Poon, Cecilia and I had met at a conference. After I had finished speaking to a large group of financial advisors, she had boldly introduced herself and offered to buy me lunch. Over our meal, I had learned that she worked as a national marketing executive with a large financial services firm in Boston. I also discovered she had always wanted to try scuba diving, one of my passions. So I passed along the names of a few dive shops in her area. I never expected to hear from her again.

To my surprise, she called each of the dive shops I had suggested and then called me to tell me about her experiences. In less than a month, she had purchased her own diving equipment and become a certified diver in the frigid waters of the North Atlantic. In my mind, this distinguished her as a risk-taker who did not just talk about her dreams. She actually made them happen. I knew that the number of female scuba divers was small compared to the number of male divers. I also knew that the number willing to dive in cold, turbulent water, male or female, was even smaller. She got my attention.

The next time I was in Boston for a speaking presentation, I contacted Cecilia. We started as diving buddies, but became fast friends. She was an intelligent and attractive woman, standing about 5 foot 4, with neatly-kept shoulder-length brown hair, blue eyes, a slim figure and an engaging personality. Despite deep Cajun roots, she had no southern drawl. Like many refined southern ladies, she carried herself with poise and confidence, and I felt instantly at ease with her. I never felt like I had to *do* anything, least of all make conversation. It simply happened naturally, as did long periods of silence as the situation dictated. This set her apart from other women I had known because she seemed to be completely comfortable with her own company and therefore could also be comfortable in mine. There was no mistaking her civility, and this stood in vivid contrast with my more rugged nature. With her palpable thirst for adventure, it almost seemed like she had been deliberately parachuted into my life for some purpose. Although I was strongly attracted to her, I never thought it would become anything serious because of the geographical distance between us. But six months after meeting her, things were starting to get more involved. I invited her to Calgary for Christmas and we decided to see if we could go scuba diving while she was there.

Anyone who lives in North America knows about winter in Canada. And every Canadian knows the lakes are frozen during that time. But Cecilia would not be deterred. After much searching, I found one lake that had open water.

Upper Waterton Lake in Waterton Lakes National Park is the deepest lake in the province of Alberta and one of the most beautiful. Straddling the Canada/U.S. border with Glacier National Park in Montana to the south, its location between jagged mountain peaks makes it a natural funnel for winds whisking through the area. It is one of the windiest places in Canada. The lake rarely freezes because most years the wind whips the waves into such a frenzy that ice can only form around the lake's edge.

It was here during a typical winter's day of bitter temperatures and

"Waterton Wind " – freezing rain being driven horizontally – that Cecilia and I graduated from being diving buddies to potential life partners.

There was at least a foot of snow on the ground. The park was all but deserted and several feet of thin ice clung to the shallow water at the lake's edge. From there, the deep, freezing-cold unknown plunged into blackness below.

Cold water scuba diving is not for the faint of heart. I suspected that if we survived the dive, our new relationship would not. Had someone asked me to bet on it, I would have wagered my life savings. Cecilia, for starters, was from Louisiana. She had grown up in Metarie, a suburb of New Orleans, below sea level. There, snow was almost an aberration. That far south, they call fifty degrees Fahrenheit "cold." I was certain, upon surfacing, that she would conclude I was a complete lunatic and exit forever from my life. Then I could go back to my vagabond and lonely existence on the road and remain single for the rest of my days.

I underestimated Cecilia.

From a rented van-turned-mobile-changing-room, we stepped into the driving wind and cold, each of us carrying sixty pounds of gear, and approached the shore with trepidation. The water temperature was only a few degrees above freezing. The wind was churning the surface of the lake into an unsettling chop. Within seconds, the freezing rain froze the hair on our foreheads into crusty mats.

Using warm and insulated dry suits and neoprene hoods to protect us from the cold, we waded slowly into the water. We carefully submerged and descended smoothly to about eighty feet. For forty magical minutes, we cruised around, gaping in awe through the crystal-clear water and immersing ourselves in the peaceful serenity of the depths. Then we resurfaced to the winter fury above.

To my amazement, Cecilia was smiling.

"That was awesome!" she squealed in delight as the frigid waves plowed into her face. "The visibility was amazing. I've never been able to see so far underwater."

I could not believe my ears.

Under the weight of our heavy gear, we struggled from the water. In an unimpressive display of self-preservation over what should have been chivalry, I hustled back to the van when I began to shiver uncontrollably.

I was just about back to the security and warmth of the vehicle when I heard a loud "thud" behind me. I turned around and saw that Cecilia had fallen face first into the snow. She was pinned there under her heavy tank and diving weights. Fearing she might suffocate, I began to sprint as well as I could back towards her.

I made it about ten feet before something astonishing happened.

Cecilia began to giggle – a small sort of giggle at first, then a laugh and ultimately, a full-blown belly roll. Within seconds, without any assistance from me, she righted herself and was back on track towards me. We embraced by the side of the van in the lee of the howling wind.

My opinion of Cecilia rocketed to the stratosphere at that moment. Not only was she strong, independent and committed, she had a buoyancy of spirit that was truly rare. I was impressed beyond description.

Within a few weeks Cecilia had declined a very high-paying promotion to Assistant Vice President with her firm and requested a one-year leave of absence to follow her heart. She moved out of her apartment in Boston's stylish Back Bay, changed countries and moved in with me in Calgary. Together, we joined forces. Cecilia became the volunteer marketer/business manager for my inspirational speaking. It proved to be a potent partnership.

Given Cecilia's happy arrival in my life, how could my emotional past be the cause of my cancer?

In the end, I realized I could go around and around on the subject of "how" forever and never reach a conclusion. The only thing I could conclude from my past was that it had become increasingly obvious over the past year that something was physically wrong. There had been a steady decline in my level of physical fitness with no change in my daily fitness regimen. Heart rate monitors do not lie. While my normal resting heart rate was usually about sixty beats a minute, it had now become an astonishing one hundred and twenty – the level of a light jog for most people. That is why I had insisted on a blood test, rather than simply antibiotics for my persistently swollen lymph glands, sore throat and loss of energy. The manufacturer of my heart rate monitor, Polar Electro, might be partially credited for helping to save my life because were it not for their device, my leukemia might have gone undetected until it was too late. I had suspected I had either mononucleosis or leukemia. I had sensed it. Now, Cecilia and I both knew.

We decided to ignore all predictions of my potential demise and give it everything we had to try to survive. We told Dr. Poon we would call in the morning to let him know when we would be ready to begin treatment.

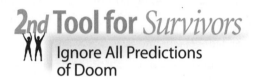

2nd Tool for *Survivors*
Ignore All Predictions of Doom

That is when we started up a mountain bigger and harder than Everest.

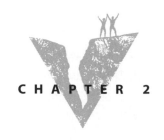

CHAPTER 2

Cecilia

A LEAP OF
FAITH

"On the other side of fear is freedom."

– Alan Hobson

Here I am, two days into a business conference in California on a bright July morning. I look at Saturday's agenda. In the 11:15 a.m. to 12:15 p.m. time slot is scheduled "motivational speaker." I say to myself, "I've seen hundreds of motivational speakers. They're all alike. I really don't need to see another one." Then conscience gets the better of me. "Now, Cecilia," it says, "you are here representing your company. You should go."

With resignation, I take an aisle seat next to a colleague in the middle of the hotel ballroom. My eyes circle the room and I make a mental note of the location of key contacts I wish to talk to at the break. I begin to plan the approach I will take with each one when I hear the introduction for the speaker. I jump in my seat as a force of energy flies by me and leaps on stage.

I look up to see a dynamic, physically fit man with intense eyes staring back at me. He stands about five foot six with blond hair, a sculpted physique and a confident presence. I feel like he is looking right at me when he speaks of his two expedition "failures." Here is this grown man in front of five hundred strangers telling everyone he cried. He instantly gains my respect. I lean forward in my chair to absorb his messages. One in particular resonates with me: "On the other side of fear is freedom. The key to unlocking the door is having the courage to take the first step."

I want to know more about how I can overcome the fears that are holding me back. Suddenly, I feel empowered. After his talk, I stand patiently at the back of the room as the long line of individuals wanting to speak with him slowly shortens. When there is no one left, I march straight up to him. I'm still thinking about his messages when I come face to face with this man who has moved me to action. I extend my hand and say, "Hi, I'm Cecilia Rau with Manulife Financial. May I buy you lunch?" I'm amazed at how bold that sounds, but I want to know more. I *have* to know more.

During lunch, Alan interviews me instead of the other way around. I find myself divulging my deepest fears to him. On the plane home, I review my notes on his presentation. I know I must learn more about managing my fears if I am to find my freedom.

Back in Boston, I go immediately to my local bookstore to purchase a copy of Alan's latest book. To my disappointment, they do not have one in stock and it will take two to three weeks to get one in. So, I phone Alan's office in Canada. His voicemail greeting says he is on the road for several speaking engagements, so I leave a message inquiring how to buy a copy of his book. Then I go to the gym. There, I hear his words in my mind as I warm up for a run on the treadmill. I recall the image in his presentation of him carrying a fifty-pound backpack on a steeply inclined treadmill. I repeat his words to myself, "CAN/WILL."

When I return home that evening, there is a message on my answering machine. I hear Alan's voice. He says he will be in Boston next week and would be happy to personally deliver a copy of his book to me. I quickly phone him back, letting him know I am most appreciative of his offer and look forward to seeing him.

Alan is to arrive at Boston's Logan airport at 7 p.m., and I anxiously await his call. But by 10 p.m., he has not phoned, so I assume his plans have changed and I prepare for bed. Then the telephone rings. An enthusiastic energized voice on the other end says, "I'm starved. Would you like to have dinner?" I hesitate for a moment, thinking it's too late to eat, but his enthusiasm overwhelms me. I find myself agreeing to meet him at his hotel.

No sooner have I entered the hotel lobby than a cheerful voice greets me. It's Alan. He has a copy of his book under his arm. It's a beautiful summer evening so we decide to walk to find a place for dinner. I apologize for not having a better knowledge of the area's restaurants as we walk by the brownstone buildings in Boston's Back Bay. Since I had only moved to the city a few months before and had been traveling extensively for my company since then, I had not eaten out very often, and especially not at this late hour.

Because most of the restaurants are closed, we end up walking around for almost an hour before we finally find a small bar that serves meals. I order a glass of wine. Alan orders a full dinner. I am amazed at his appetite. I think to myself, "How can someone so lean and fit eat so much so late at night?" I surely can't.

During dinner, Alan autographs his book for me. I express my desire to learn to scuba dive, not confessing that I haven't taken a course because I'm afraid to fail.

One week after my dinner with Alan, I am on my dream vacation – two weeks at a horse ranch in Wyoming. I ride each day, go whitewater rafting for the first time and hike in the Grand Tetons. When I leave the ranch I declare, "I'll be back to be a guide next summer." I hope to keep that promise. To do so, I'll have to step outside my comfort zone and face my fears of taking a risk and doing something new.

It won't be the first time I've done so. My move to Boston was a big leap. I had spent thirty-eight years in New Orleans, attending college near home and working for Manulife there so I could care for my father after my mother's death from breast cancer when I was 18. When I was offered a position in the company's U.S. head office in Boston, I hoped I could use the knowledge and experience I'd gained in the field to create changes at the corporate level and benefit others. After much deliberation, I accepted the position. Then I had the uncomfortable task of telling my father. Because he never re-married after my mother's death, I felt a great responsibility to him. He was sad I was leaving.

After the trip to Wyoming, returning to Boston and the office is difficult. I think about my time in the West and question why I am living in a city when my passion is for the outdoors. At the end of my first week back, I feel drained of energy as I walk back to my studio apartment. When I get home, I check my voicemail and there is Alan's dynamic voice again, giving me a list of some of the scuba diving shops in the Boston area. I pick up the phone and call the nearest one. A man answers on the first ring. I tell him I'm interested in learning to dive. I discover there is a class the next day. "Okay," I say, "sign me up."

For the first time since my trip to Wyoming, I go to bed that night feeling good about myself. The next morning, I'm a little apprehensive. As I drive to the dive shop, I tell myself, "I CAN do this. I WILL do this."

Two weeks later, I'm a certified diver. Proudly, I phone Alan to thank him for his encouragement and tell him of my accomplishment. I have even purchased my own diving equipment and I'm raring to dive. To my surprise, he says he will be in the Boston area in two weeks for a speaking presentation and he'll bring his diving gear.

I eagerly await his arrival. I have everything ready. The van is rented, the air tanks reserved. I even have directions to a dive shop in Cape Ann, a rocky head of land on the ocean north of Boston.

On the drive to Cape Ann, we are like two kids playing hooky from school, giddy with the excitement of an outing together. I'm able to find out a little more about him – where he lives in Canada, who his family members are and what food and movies he likes. We are both comfortable with silence, and we spend long stretches quietly taking in the scenery along the way.

Over the next few months, we have the opportunity to dive together several times. Each outing brings us closer together emotionally, but geographically, we are thousands of miles apart. It is during one of our dive trips that I realize Alan is more than a good friend and dive buddy. He is the love of my life.

The discovery is sudden. As we come around a turn on the narrow winding road on the way to our favorite dive spot, a horse gallops out of nowhere right in front of the vehicle. Alan quickly brakes. We are both stunned for a moment, our mouths open. Without hesitation, Alan pulls over, gets out of the van and begins to follow the horse on foot, hoping to guide it away from the busy street. In the process, he is almost trampled by several other horses. They seem to have escaped their paddock.

Soon, a middle-aged man and woman with halters in hand come running up to us. I let them know the direction in which the first horse has run and then I follow them up a hill. Alan and I help them look for their horses for almost an hour. Finally, we find one of the animals grazing on a large patch of grass in a nearby yard. The rest are still loose.

Thankful to have been able to recover at least one of the horses, we return to the van. I find myself overwhelmed with feelings of admiration and love for Alan. Seeing him take action on behalf of a stranger sends a surge of warmth through me. It is a sensation I have never experienced before. My feelings for him leap to another level.

We manage to see each other a few times during the fall. One day Alan asks if I would like to spend Christmas with him in Canada. I jump at the chance. Of course, I insist we go diving together. Even though it's winter, he manages to find a good place.

Our Christmas together is magical. My fortieth birthday falls during the holiday and to celebrate, Alan surprises me with a dogsled ride in Banff National Park. I find myself driving a team of Huskies with the cold wind blowing in my face and the sun on my back. We glide up and down hills laughing like children. I feel so alive.

Our relationship blossoms during that visit. At the airport when it comes time to leave, I am joyful about the time we have had together and sad because it has come to an end. With mixed feelings, I board the plane.

Back in Boston, I find myself thinking often of Alan. I look around my office and out the window at the building next door. I long for the beauty of the Canadian Rockies. Early in the New Year, while attending a North American sales meeting in Toronto, the Vice President of Sales offers me a major promotion to Assistant Vice President and informs me that the announcement will be made the next morning. I'm stunned at the news. I have worked hard to earn this promotion, yet for some reason I feel uneasy about accepting it. I am an individual who commits one hundred percent to whatever I am doing, but I need to feel passionately about what I am doing. If I accept this promotion, I fear it will mean more travel and less of a life for *me*.

I ask myself a question: "Am I making a difference in my current job?" Then I ask another: "Will I make more of a difference if I accept the promotion?" The answer to both questions is "no."

Suddenly, I know what I must do. I must make a leap of faith. I must face my fears of the unknown. I must find my freedom. So I not only turn down the position, but ask for a one-year leave of absence too. For the first time since coming to Boston, I do something for me.

The next day, I call Alan to tell him the news. He asks me what I'm going to do. When I tell him I'm not sure, he presses me. "Cecilia," he says. "I've not known you a long time, but I've known you long enough to know that you always have a pretty good idea of what you're going to do next. So, what's next?"

"I want to move to Canada and live with you," I say.

Two and a half months later, I take off for a new life full of adventure. On the flight to Calgary, I review in my mind the changes that have taken place in my life. I have always worked, even during college. I have always defined myself by what I did. Now, without a job, I will have to define myself by who I am. That's a big question: "Who am I?"

I guess I'm about to find out.

CHAPTER 3

Alan
TAKING THE FIRST STEP

"It's not what you have. It's what you do with what you have."

– John Hughes,
Around-the-World Solo Ocean Sailor,
One Step Beyond

I feel like I'm suffocating. Every breath is a battle. I look at my altimeter. It reads 27,600 feet. Camp 4 is a long way below me. If I fall here, I'm history. I'll slide all the way into the South Col and maybe 4,000 feet down the Lhotse Face too. Everest in all its massiveness will consume me like a crumb.

If I could just get to the ridge. If I could somehow just get there. Maybe we'd stand a chance. Are we off route? Why can't I keep up?...

I feel alone and very, very afraid…

I took a step. It seemed to feel okay, so I took another, then another and another. I thought, 'Well, if I'm able to move, maybe I'll be able to warm up. If I'm able to warm up, maybe, just maybe, I'll be able to keep from freezing to death on this mountain.'

It's fascinating in life to see what happens to us when we take a

few steps. Because we're off balance and in motion, we take a few
more...and a few more. Pretty soon, if we can somehow stay on our
feet, we start to cover ground, we break through our self-doubt and
fear and we begin to discover one of the ultimate truths of life:
    On the other side of fear is freedom.

–From Everest to Enlightenment

I felt torn between two states. Emotionally, I was inert. The only sensation was a vacuous numbness. Mentally, my mind was racing like the point of a laser beam blasting at light speed across the galaxy. The psychologists call this state post-traumatic shock. It is supposed to be one of the ways the body protects itself during intense stress.

Cecilia insisted I speak immediately with my parents and three brothers. That was the last thing I wanted to do. I just wanted to crawl under a rock and disappear.

She would not hear of it.

"If anyone in your family had cancer, they'd tell you right away," she said emphatically. "You owe it to them."

How do you tell your parents that a child they love might predecease them? Given my parents' previous experience with my two nephews, I feared they might take my news hard.

I was wrong.

"How do you spell the name of this condition?" my mother asked stoically. "Can you ask the doctors if your condition might be related to either of the two different conditions your nephews had?"

I agreed, described my illness as simply as I could and tried to put a positive spin on my diagnosis. I explained that the prognosis looked reasonably good and that it looked even better if an adult blood stem cell or bone marrow donor could be found. I did not tell them that the average three-year survival rate for patients with acute myeloid leukemia was only fifteen percent. Thankfully, I did not know that then. Dr. Poon, I would discover months later, had been very careful not to stress the subtle but critically important difference between remission and survival. He had explained it at the time of my diagnosis, but I had not heard it. My thoughts had been elsewhere.

My father, a research scientist who typically focused only on the facts, responded as he usually did – with supportive self-control. "Sounds very difficult, Son, but we're here for you any time of the day or night. Let us know just as soon as you know more. We'll be waiting."

I was not able to reach any of my brothers, so I left each of them a carefully worded telephone message.

Surprisingly, those were not the toughest calls to make. One of the toughest was to my agents at the Washington Speakers Bureau in Virginia. The Washington Speakers Bureau is widely acknowledged as one of the finest speakers bureaus in the world. To be represented by them is like being called up to the majors in baseball or being drafted into the NBA. They represent everyone from Margaret Thatcher to Rudy Giuliani. The problem was, my relationship with them was only ninety days old. I hardly knew them, or they me.

Almost as much as I feared cancer, I feared bankruptcy. I was terrified the bureau might drop me like a stone and move on to represent another Everest summiteer. Then, not only would I be sick, I would have no income either. Even with Cecilia as my volunteer sales and marketing director, if I were ill, there would be little for her to market.

The bureau's reaction was impressive. The two founding partners, Bernie Swain and Harry Rhoads, Jr., immediately asked when I wanted them to fly out to see me. One of the senior agents, Michael Menchel, swiftly sent us a touching note. They too had experienced cancer in their past, as had some of the other speakers they represented. "You will survive this," they said insistently, "and when you do, you will be an even better presenter because of it. We'll be with you all the way. Just let us know when you're ready to speak again. We'll block off the calendar for as long as you need."

Next, Cecilia and I briefed the staff that ran my office. They too took the news well.

"You survived three Everest expeditions," they affirmed resolutely. "You can survive this too."

Cecilia and I went home to our apartment that night reassured, but still very undecided about what to do. We sat at the kitchen table and discussed the options. Should we try only conventional medicine, or complementary or alternative medicine, or should we just resign ourselves to fate? We were supposed to have committed to chemotherapy, but clearly we had not yet fully.

Sometime during the wee small hours, we ran out of talk and fell asleep. When we awakened, we had run out of time.

Later that morning, we called Dr. Poon and asked to be admitted. Within ninety minutes, he had secured me a bed in the Special Services Building of Calgary's Foothills Medical Centre, a treatment facility adjoining the Tom Baker Cancer Centre where I had received my diagnosis. My first session of week-long, twenty-four-hour chemotherapy would begin the next day.

On this mountain, there was only one way to find out if there really was freedom on the other side of fear. We had to remove the doubt and go find out. So hand in hand, shaking, but still roped together, Cecilia and I prepared to take our first frightening steps into the unknown.

▼

The puja ceremony was spectacular. The entire team was decked out in our bright yellow, red and black Sun Ice one-piece climbing suits. They stood out sharply against the white snow backdrop and brilliant blue sky of base camp. Under a slight breeze, birds swooped and darted here and there over the hand-built stone altar the Sherpas had constructed over the previous days. As wave after wave of sweet-smelling smoke from the burning of juniper boughs twisted and turned its way skyward from the altar, the local monk's chants created a scene of stirring spiritualism.

It is forbidden for any climbing team to set foot on Everest without a puja ceremony. The Sherpas believe that you must ask permission to tread upon Chomolungma's skin and that to ascend to the summit without such license is tantamount to violating the Mother Goddess in the most intimate way. Whether you believe in such things or not is immaterial. What is material is that you respect the culture and spirituality of the Sherpas.

I decided I'd do anything the Sherpas asked me to do. This was, after all, their mountain.

– From Everest to Enlightenment

Cecilia and I gathered up a few things from our apartment, stuffed them into one of the backpacks I had used on Everest, and headed to my office a block away to finish packing. At my request, she recorded our journey to the hospital with a video camera. Because my parents were on the other side of the country, I thought that the closer we could bring them to our situation, the less anxious they might feel. Perhaps a videotape of my treatment would help. I also felt that if this was to be the beginning of my last days on Earth, I wanted some way to make a final statement. So while our office assistant, Tracy Wuth, helped me fill the remaining space in my backpack with a small television/VCR, laptop computer, herbal supplements and a few books, Cecilia videotaped. Incredibly, she somehow found the composure to do it. When all was ready, we loaded my gear into Tracy's truck and the three of us got in.

Our first stop was a nearby Thai restaurant for a final taste of "real" food before I was subjected to the gastronomical delights of hospital fare. I would have devoured the tasty buffet but I really did not have much of an appetite.

We said little over lunch, at least little of any significance. I remember what a glorious summer day it was. The sun's warm rays streamed in through the restaurant windows, but I felt nothing but cold. It was like sitting on the edge of a glacial crevasse with the frigid air blowing up at me from the icy abyss below. It chilled me deeply.

When we were finished, we stood, paid our bill and returned to Tracy's vehicle. The drive to the hospital was fifteen minutes at most, and it was over too fast. Despite my condition, I was in no hurry to arrive.

I had a harsh, dark view of hospitals. I did not believe they were places of healing. They were places of treatment. If you wanted to get better, you had to get the heck out of there as soon as your treatment was over. My deepest desire from the beginning of treatment was to get to the end of it as quickly as possible. That way, I felt I had a chance. I believed this to the depth of my soul. I was like a caged tiger pacing impatiently. From the moment I walked in, I wanted to walk out. If they took my body to the morgue after I was discharged, that was one thing, but I was not going to die in a hospital. I drew the line there.

Cecilia and I went straight to the admitting department as instructed by Dr. Poon's office. I walked up to the clerk at the window, told her my name and pulled out my blue provincial healthcare card. Within seconds, she found my name on the hospital's computer, waved the screen with an electronic wand to let it know I had arrived, and handed me a piece of paper.

"This is a consent-to-treatment form," she said pleasantly. "Please fill it in and sign it."

"Thank you," I said, sitting down.

I stopped when I came to a question about the type of room I wanted.

"It says here I can choose between a public room and a private one," I said to the admitting clerk, "but you have to pay extra for a private one."

"That's right," she said, "but you're going to Unit 57. On Unit 57, private rooms are free to patients."

Great, I thought to myself. Thank goodness for public healthcare.

Unit 57, I would learn, was the acute care ward for cancer patients. Private rooms were free for those who needed them when the effects of radiation and chemotherapy suppressed patients' immune systems so significantly that each *had* to have a private room or risk dying from infection by fellow patients, staff or visitors. So although "free" sounded good, it only sounded good if you were not actually being admitted to Unit 57.

When the paperwork was completed a few minutes later, Cecilia and I got into the elevator beside the admitting area. When we got to the fifth floor, we walked up to the nursing station and introduced ourselves.

"Yes, Mr. Hobson," one of the nurses replied brightly. "We've been waiting for you. Your bed is ready and we'll take you straight there."

Still half hoping all this was nothing but a big mistake, Cecilia and I looked at each other, deflated.

Suddenly, a colorfully dressed nurse with an equally effervescent personality appeared before us.

"Hello, Alan and Cecilia, my name is Kim Newhouse. I'm going to be your nurse this evening. I'm going to help you get started."

Kim took one look at my backpack, smiled and said, "My, that's quite a load you have there. You look like you're leaving on an expedition. Dr. Poon told us to expect an adventurer, but we didn't expect him to show up with his tent and sleeping bag."

Cecilia and I laughed. It broke the tension.

Kim escorted us to a room at the end of the hall. Along the way, we peered hesitantly into the other cubicles. We saw adult patients of every age and description, some in hospital gowns, some awake, others sleeping, some entertaining visitors. Most were hooked up to I.V. poles, many with multiple bags hanging from them. The doors to some rooms were closed. Signs affixed to them indicated that no one could enter without first washing their hands.

My room, like the others, was remarkably colorful. The door and clothes closet were bright red. The window faced west towards the distant Rocky Mountains. I could not actually see them, but I did have a very pleasant view of the Bow River valley several hundred feet below. Although no hospital room could be described as upbeat, this one was a long way from dismal.

"Could we turn the bed around so I could see out the window?" I asked.

"We might be able to do that, Alan, but it could take a bit of jury-rigging," Kim replied. "All the oxygen, suction and other systems usually need to be close to the patient's head. If we turn your bed around, all that essential stuff will be at your feet."

"Believe me, Kim, after you smell my feet, you'll be the one needing the oxygen."

We laughed again, thankfully.

The very fact that Kim was willing to work with us on how to position the bed impressed us. We would discover that just about any reasonable request was considered on Unit 57. Although I had previously believed hospital wards were rigid, impersonal places, I was about to learn that this ward was different. The nurses here were specially trained in acute care. Extra staff was added to provide a higher level of attention twenty-four hours a day, and there was an understanding that patients there might not have a lot of time left.

Kim was a superb nurse. Although she looked young enough to be in her late twenties, her interpersonal skills and maturity belied her youthful appearance. She explained in great detail what we could expect in the coming hours and weeks, how I might feel, how the ward worked and what amenities were available to us in the form of kitchen facilities, exercise equipment and reading materials. She swiftly, thoroughly and pleasantly answered our every question, not only with a ream of invaluable medical information, but with a confidence that put us at ease. She had the situation under control.

Then a light entered the room. My long-time friend and physiotherapist, Patti Mayer, swept in. Patti had brilliant blue eyes, short blonde hair and round rosy cheeks. She never went anywhere at half speed. She was energetic and vital and she moved with a spring in her step and a mission in her heart. She wanted to positively affect every person with whom she came in contact.

Patti had followed my gradual physical deterioration closely during the previous months and when the diagnosis finally came, outside of my family, she had been one of the first people I told.

"I've come to spiritually bless and cleanse your room," she announced matter-of-factly.

Patti had my complete trust. She had successfully treated many of the physical injuries I had experienced while training for my adventure expeditions. In addition to being a gifted physiotherapist, in recent years she had expanded her knowledge to include acupuncture, Chinese medicine, the ancient Chinese art of Qi Gong (energy building), the Japanese practice of Reiki (energy movement), herbal medicines, vitamins and other forms of complementary and alternative healing. She now worked regularly with cancer patients and her expertise was surpassed only by her spirit. She meditated daily, and when she walked into our room, she did so with such buoyancy you would swear she was there to attend a wedding.

In a way she was. Patti had come to witness a marriage of western and complementary medicine custom-made for me. While the nurses and doctors worked to treat my body using western medical techniques, she was there to treat my soul. She brought with her a stuffed animal, a beautiful beige-colored puppy we named "Happy." We immediately placed him on guard duty at the head of my bed. Then we left the room briefly so she could do her work.

Surprisingly, the staff seemed fine with Patti's presence.

"Whatever works for you and will help you get better works for us," Kim said confidently, "as long as we know what you're doing so we don't work at cross-purposes with each other."

The nurses had obviously been down this road before. Gone, apparently, were the days when western medicine prohibited any other form of treatment. In my mind, this established Unit 57 as a facility of strength. It was not rigid and controlling, but open to other ideas and concepts. Whether this acceptance was ward policy or simply our good fortune, we did not know, but at that moment we did not care. From that time forward, every complementary healer we brought into my room and every unorthodox method I used were accepted as long as we kept all caregivers informed.

From a psychological perspective, this made the prospect of chemotherapy seem much less threatening. We could see that as uncomfortable as my treatment was likely to be, and as frightened as we were, we could feel at home on 57 – even if I could not wait to leave.

So Cecilia and I began to build a team around us, creating a personalized blend of medical professionals, including anything and anyone we felt could help.

Patti had no sooner finished her blessing than we learned the next rule of life on 57 – it was always changing. Kim announced that I was to move to the room across the hall so that a more critically ill patient might receive radiation in the room I was occupying. The room I was in had walls, floor and ceiling lined with lead. This permitted the in-room radiation of patients too ill to be moved to the basement of the hospital where radiation therapy usually took place.

Without a word of complaint, Patti went immediately across the hall, repeated her work there and within minutes declared that all was ready. So Cecilia, Patti, Kim and I packed up my clothes and grabbed the television. We took the Tibetan prayer flags I had purchased the last time I had been in Kathmandu and a few other spiritual items. One was a framed picture of a point of light I use for meditation.

Once we had settled in, Patti called me into the hall.

"I have to go now," she said softly, "but I'll be back soon, my friend, probably tomorrow. Things will be all right, Alan. There is great care here. I feel it."

Then she hugged me and whispered in my ear. "You will teach them more than they will teach you," she said knowingly. "Just be who you are. They will see, and so will you."

After a gentle kiss on the cheek, she left.

That night, they took me down to radiology and put a catheter in my chest. It was designed to mainline the chemotherapy straight into my heart and from there directly into my bloodstream. The line would stay embedded for over six months. With the help of a local anesthetic, I was conscious and pain-free throughout the procedure. I chatted freely with the technicians and interventional radiologist who did the work.

"So how'd it go?" Cecilia asked when they wheeled me out afterwards on a gurney. "It seemed like you were in there forever."

"Hardly felt it," I said. "These guys are pros."

When we got back to my room, Kim was there to greet us.

"You might have some difficulty sleeping tonight," she explained. "The central line is bound to be a bit uncomfortable at first. If it gets to be too much, just call the nursing station and your night nurse can bring you a painkiller.

"Congratulations, Alan. You've cleared the first hurdle. Now we'll give you a while to rest. Chemo starts first thing tomorrow. This probably feels as if it's all coming at you like a bullet train."

Then she turned to leave.

"As you go, Kim," I said, "could you blow on that prayer flag hanging from the television? When you do, the prayer printed on it will be sent up to the Mother Goddess to ask for my safe passage to the summit and back again."

She smiled kindly.

"Of course," she said.

With a puff and a flutter, the first prayer went skyward as Kim left the room.

Cecilia crawled into bed with me for a snuggle. It was wonderful to have her there. I knew that this experience was either going to deepen our relationship or end it. At that moment, there was no way of knowing which way it was going to go. In fact, there was no way of knowing which way any of this was going to go.

As I lay there in a state of partial shock, I tried to digest the day's experiences. This really was looking more and more like a Himalayan expedition. We had had a little puja ceremony with our "monk," Patti; there were Sherpa nurses, doctor guides, prayer flags, other climbers and an uncertain outcome. I was apprehensive, a little queasy and definitely finding it difficult acclimatizing to my new environment.

What a humbling day it had been. Alan Hobson, "Mt. Everest Climber & Summiteer," was now a cancer patient in a hospital bed. I had to park my ego, discard my previous identity and conserve my energy for the long climb ahead. Somehow, I had to surrender to the process and the plan. My objective, however, was crystal clear: get up, get going and get back on top.

As I guarded the strange central line dangling uncomfortably from my chest, I did my best to hold Cecilia. Awkwardly, we drifted off to a fitful sleep.

Base camp had been established.

CHAPTER 4

Cecilia

A HARD FALL

In August in Calgary, the evenings are warm, the air is filled with the scent of lilacs and the sun doesn't set until well after 9 p.m. It's my favorite time for a bike ride. There are hundreds of miles of bike paths along the Bow River. The icy waters run clear and the fly fishermen can be seen along the banks casting for elusive trout. All species of waterfowl flock to the water's edge.

I share the paths with the active residents of Calgary, some on roller blades, some running, others on bikes pulling child carriers, many walking their dogs. Hand in hand, stride by stride, children of all ages are enjoying the carefree days of summer.

I smile and wave, acknowledging the pure joy of being outdoors as I pass others on the pathway. Everyone is careful to dodge our beautiful Canada geese who are tough and stand their ground. I often see cyclists and runners queued in wait for the geese and their goslings as they waddle across the pathway. This is all part of summer in Calgary.

But that was last August. No longer am I among the active people on the pathways. Alan and I are no longer enjoying the warm summer evenings. We have lost our freedom to cancer.

I hate having the word "cancer" back in my vocabulary. The mere mention of it knocks me numb. I remember as a child climbing our hundred-year-old oak tree in the backyard in New Orleans. I was so proud of how high I had climbed. I was up to the third level of branches when all of a sudden I lost my hold and fell to the ground. I hit hard. The wind was knocked out of me. For what seemed like an eternity, I couldn't breathe, I couldn't call for help and I couldn't move. I could only lie there helplessly until the air returned to my lungs. That's how the word cancer makes me feel. It takes my breath away.

Saying the word makes it real. I am sitting in my office, reaching for the phone. I stare at the number pad. What is the telephone number of the Washington Speakers Bureau? I have dialed it a hundred times. I know it like my own, but for some reason, I can't seem to remember it now.

"Start with the area code, Cecilia," I talk myself through. "Start with the first number."

Hesitantly, I press 7. It breaks the barrier.

A friendly voice answers, "Good afternoon. This is Karen. May I help you?" I immediately reply with a pleasant, "Good afternoon, Karen. May I speak with Michael Menchel?" I hope nothing in my voice gives me away.

Michael's greeting is warm and enthusiastic as always. I feel myself relaxing in my chair, my mind searching for the right words. I take a deep breath and say, "Alan has cancer and has been diagnosed with leukemia. They will start treatment right away. We will have to reschedule his speaking engagements for the next six months."

There, I've said it. I've said the words "Alan has cancer." Until now, it has just been a bad dream.

Michael's voice is full of compassion and support. I assure him that Alan will be speaking again soon. The first call is made, so I move to the next. Each call brings cancer closer.

It becomes even more real two days later when I not only say it, but see it. On Unit 57, people are walking their I.V. poles down the corridors, committed caregivers by their sides. Many patients are bald. I enjoy smiling at the patients and their caregivers to see if I can elicit a smile in return. Some try to smile. You can see the corners of their lips turn up a little, but the twinkle that was once in their eyes is now dim. I smile anyway. It makes me feel better.

Our orientation begins with a walk around the unit. One of the nurses, Kim Newhouse, gives us the tour. She takes us past the nurses' station – the command zone and heart of the unit. Adjacent to the command zone is the "war room." The war room has a large white board on one wall. Names and numbers are written in bold black, red and green ink, along with plus and minus signs. Kim explains that this is where the nurses begin and end their shifts. They record which patients are doing well and which ones are not. The enemy is cancer, the ammunition is care. These acute care nurses have seen the best and worst in battle. They have endured many wars.

We walk towards the only natural light at the end of the hall. Stopping before we reach its warmth, Kim points out the "Quiet Room." This room is for patients and loved ones to talk or use the phone in private. I comment how nice it is to have a quiet place to go, to escape the noise of the unit. I look in. The walls are a pale blue, and there are two large upholstered chairs, a small table with a phone and a box of tissues next to it. My eyes are drawn to the plaques and photographs on the walls. They are memorials for deceased loved ones who have spent time on Unit 57. A chill runs through me. I turn away. This is not a place of tranquility as I first thought. It is not a place of comfort. It is a place of sorrow where people call friends and family members to tell them of the diagnosis or the latest prognosis. I will find other phones to use, phones in well-lit areas. I don't like the closed-in feel of the Quiet Room. I will not spend much time there.

We turn from the chill of the Quiet Room and enter the common area. Large windows let in the afternoon sunlight. Now this is a place I like. The patients and caregivers are bathed in sunlight. A mother is playing cards with her young daughter who is hooked up to an I.V. pole. An older gentleman is working on a crossword puzzle as he takes a break from his bedside station. A woman works on a cross-stitch pattern awaiting the return of her husband from his latest test. Here is activity, here is life within the hospital walls.

We leave the common area and walk a few feet down the hall. I try not to look into the patients' rooms as we walk past, but my curiosity is strong. I can't help but peer in to see how others are doing. I see lots of balloons, but no flowers. There are many photographs and lots of cards on the walls. I think how lovely it would be to have some fresh flowers. When I ask Kim why the only place I see flowers is at the nurses' station, she says, "We will talk about that later. Let's continue the tour for now." "Okay," I say in an uncertain tone. I have so much to learn.

We shuffle down the hall and come to the unit's bulletin board. The brown corkboard is filled with messages. I stop to read one, "When you get to the end of your rope, tie a knot and hang on. The situation is temporary." I will come back here often to read many of these inspirational messages. I will even post my own.

Next on the tour is the kitchen. I think, how wonderful, they have all the conveniences of home, even a kitchen equipped with two large refrigerators, toaster, microwave and blender. It's really nice to have all of these amenities for our brief stay here.

Little do I know that my opinion will soon change.

CHAPTER 5

Alan
INTO THE
ICEFALL

*"The scariest thing was the night before, lying at the bottom
of the climb and trying to sleep, knowing that the next day,
you'd be going up there. You camp at the bottom and look up
at this bloody great precipice going into the sky and wonder
what it's going to be like up there. But you don't know.
That's the time when you're most tempted
to turn around and go home."*

– John Amatt,
Climber/Adventurer,
One Step Beyond

On April 15, Jason, five of our climbing Sherpas and I headed
into the darkness of the Khumbu Icefall at 4 a.m. The Icefall is a glacier
that gets squeezed between Everest on one side and its sister peak, Mt.
Nuptse, on the other. It tumbles 2,000 feet over a rock ledge and in the
process splits into ice blocks the size of hotels. The whole thing is in
constant motion, often moving up to several feet a day. On any other
mountain you would never go in here. It is simply too dangerous. But
on the southern, Nepalese side of Everest, if you hope to make it to the

summit you have to go in here. There is no other route to the top.

That morning the icefall was as it usually was – a mind-boggling labyrinth of crevasses, ice blocks, ladders and anxiety, especially by headlamp...

The first time I crossed one of the ladders spanning a crevasse, I was petrified. With only a single strand of limp, quarter-inch thick climbing rope on which to hold with each hand, I had to carefully ensure my crampons – those spikes on the bottoms of my boots used to give me purchase in the ice and snow – were placed exactly on the 10-inch-spaced rungs of the ladder, step by tentative step. As I am not very fond of heights, I was somewhat relieved to realize that in the dark I couldn't see the bottom of the crevasse. There were at least 15 stories, or about 150 feet, beneath the soles of my boots...

As I gingerly made my way across the ladder, under the weight of my body, the ladder began to bow, swaying up and down and creaking with a terrifying sound. Periodically, gusts of wind would buffet me from side to side. To prevent myself from pitching sideways into the crevasse, I squeezed the safety lines like they were life itself.

The steel points of my crampons dug sharply into the soft aluminum rungs, sometimes holding my feet momentarily as I tried to bring them carefully forward. Up and down, side to side, forward and back I swayed. The whole experience was unnerving. I seriously contemplated crawling. But I was an Everest climber. They don't crawl! Crawling was for babies. I may have felt like one, but I could overcome this.

"You CAN, Alan," I told myself. "You WILL."

Some of the ladder bridges were four and five sections across – a horizontal distance of 50 or 60 feet. They were lashed together with rope. It was pitch black, freezing cold, my heart was racing, my chest was heaving and my legs felt like rubber. My whole body began to quiver. It was all I could do to keep from shaking myself right into the blackness below...

I learned a powerful lesson crossing those ladders in the Icefall, one that I continue to use today. To cross the ladders you had to look down. You had to see where you were placing your feet. In looking down you had a choice of where you looked – as far as the rungs of the ladder or way the hell down into that terrifyingly deep hole beyond.

So often in life we focus on the hole – on all those terrible things that could happen to us, on all those things outside our control, when the only things we should be focusing on are those things within our control – the tiny steps we need to take this minute to get us to where we want to go.

– From Everest to Enlightenment

Sometime during the early morning hours of August 12, I said a little prayer. Although I am not a religious man, I am a spiritual one, and my years in the mountains had taught me to respect a Higher Power. For the past few years I had practiced a form of meditation called Raja Yoga. It was designed to silence the mind, soothe the soul and improve one's ability to stay focused on the present. Unlike other forms of yoga, it does not involve stretching, special breathing or mantras. And it is done with the eyes open. The primary objective is to manage the mind, not only while meditating, but also throughout daily activities. Meditation creates connection with an inner peace and with the inestimable power and intellect of a Supreme Soul called "Baba," the Father.

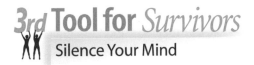

3rd Tool for *Survivors*
Silence Your Mind

"Please, Baba," I prayed, "send me your best man."

He did. And he was, appropriately, a woman.

Rita Dillabough appeared at my bedside at 7:30 a.m. sharp. She had short, dark hair, a warm engaging smile and a soft, sweet voice. Her touch was light and soothing, and she moved as effortlessly around the room as she would around her own living room. Her glasses encircled eyes that twinkled brightly, and they instantly communicated compassion and care. From the moment we met her, Cecilia and I knew she had been divinely sent. My prayer had been answered.

"Good morning, Alan," she said smiling as she introduced herself. "I hope you and Cecilia got at least some sleep. Breakfast will be along shortly, but first we have some preparations to make."

Rita immediately began a long lesson in Chemotherapy 101: which drugs I would receive, what side effects to expect and how I might feel. She did this with a tranquil confidence that could only come from years of experience. Around her neck was a stethoscope, in one of the pockets of her smock was a pad of paper and pen, and around her wrist was a watch she used to keep track of all infusions, injections and other important medical data she would later enter into my medical chart. She wore standard-issue turquoise hospital fatigues covered with a brightly colored hospital smock. Like all good nurses, she was a stickler for detail, procedure and precision. Given the strength of some of the medications she was administering, the severity of the illnesses many of the patients on the ward were experiencing and the level of care some of them required, this was no surprise. To us, it was also reassuring. We knew we were in good hands.

Rita was no stranger to challenge. Married, with four children, she lived on a rural acreage a short distance from town. She had two children still living at home, as well as horses, dogs, cats, cattle and a rugged, straight-shooting husband, Brian, who worked in the oil service industry. Both Rita and Brian had grown up on farms. Rita was used to multi-tasking, meeting the demands of a busy family and rising on "work" days at 5 a.m. for a 7 a.m. start at the hospital where she worked part-time.

She explained that I would be receiving what some doctors called a "three-and-seven" – one drug daily for three days and the other drug at the same time for seven days. The first drug, a red substance called idarubicin, would be injected into my central line each morning, while the second medication, a clear liquid called cytarabine, would be infused intravenously around-the-clock. The first round of chemotherapy, she explained, was called "induction chemo."

While I listened to Rita, Cecilia took notes. Although most of the terms were Greek to me, her internet research had prepared her well. She looked like she was back at university, except that the intensity in her eyes revealed a purpose beyond the academic. It was good to know she was there, because although I listened as intently as I could, I had reached intellectual and emotional overload days earlier.

The theory behind chemotherapy is relatively simple. It is designed to kill all rapidly reproducing cells, especially cancer cells. Unfortunately, it also kills any rapidly reproducing healthy cells like those that make up the roots of human hair. That is why patients receiving chemo usually lose their hair. It is a positive sign: tangible evidence the medicine is working.

The chemotherapy I was to receive had been specifically chosen to kill the rapidly reproducing immature white blood cells in my bloodstream. At the same time, however, it would destroy most of my mature white blood cells, red blood cells and platelets. The longer I received this kind of chemo, the less energy I would have, the more vulnerable I would be to uncontrolled internal or external bleeding and the less resistance I would have to disease. My disease-fighting cells, my mature white blood cells, would be almost eliminated.

Chemo seemed to me like a controlled fall into a glacial crevasse. Each day that goes by, patients slide further down a slippery slope. They feel weaker and weaker until finally, about a week or two after the chemo has stopped flowing, they hit the bottom of the crevasse. Like climbers at high altitude, they do not eat well (if at all), sleep well or feel well. It is like growing old very fast.

After hitting bottom, the body takes time to recover – at least three to six weeks in most cases. When the levels of red blood cells, white blood cells and platelets in the blood have rebounded somewhat, a bone marrow biopsy is done to see if any cancer cells are still present. If they are – and for added "insurance" even if they are not – patients usually undergo successive waves of chemotherapy. These waves continue until the cancer cells cannot be detected anymore. Immature white blood cells – cancerous blast cells – are not strong enough to withstand these waves. But normal, healthy cells are usually far more resilient. This is the key to chemotherapy.

The treatment works as long as the patients and their normal cells can withstand it. The problem is, after repeated waves of the medicine, even healthy cells lose their resilience. The result is that patients can die, not from cancer, but from complications arising from chemo. Herein lies the delicate balance between life and death, not only for cancer cells, but also for patients.

Ideally, the cancer goes into remission with as few waves of chemotherapy as possible. This does not necessarily mean the cancer is gone. It simply means that for the moment, the number of cancer cells in the body is below a detectable level. Up to an astonishing ten billion cancer cells may still remain, but not be clinically detectable. If they are not detectable, the cancer is said to be "in remission." If patients stay in remission for at least five years, they are generally considered cured.

In my case, Dr. Poon was aiming for that "cure." If he was able to put my leukemia into remission, an adult blood stem cell or bone marrow transplant might, if all went well, eradicate the disease from my body. Then, provided that I showed no symptoms of the disease for five years, I might be cured.

I had to cross this crevasse. Along the way, any number of things could go wrong. The side effects of chemo could kill me or my leukemia could. It was like setting foot for the first time in the deadly Khumbu Icefall – I could plummet into a bottomless slot, a huge ice block might collapse from above and crush me, or I could be swept away by a sudden avalanche. There was risk everywhere.

Rita knew this. And after her careful explanation, so did we.

"Just one more thing before we begin," she said.

She handed me a little yellow pill.

"This is Zofran," she announced. "It's an anti-nauseant. You should take one every eight hours."

"Wonderful," I said. "Let's hope it works."

"Oh, it usually does," she asserted. "The research done by pharmaceutical companies has come a long way in recent years. Generally, chemo patients experience a lot less nausea than in the past thanks to the new anti-nauseant medications and their use in combinations. This can make a huge difference to the quality of life for patients during treatment."

"Great," I blurted. "Let's give it a go."

Quickly, I downed the pill, winking at Cecilia as reassuringly as I could.

Next Rita brought me a cup of crushed ice.

"Many chemo patients find that extra fluids help reduce the nausea," she explained. "We're going to encourage you to drink lots of water so you stay cool and well hydrated. Good hydration helps flush out the chemo and toxins created by the death of the cancer cells in your body."

Patti Mayer had told me that during chemotherapy, the body experiences an excess release of heat. In Chinese medicine, this is called "yang," or male energy. For the body to recover from chemo, this heat has to be counter-balanced by cooler "yin," or female energy. This can be done through meditation, special breathing, or being outdoors in nature. Another way is to drink water constantly. This helps rebalance the body's internal energy and put out its chemical "fires." It also increases the frequency of urination which helps purge the body of the powerful medicine once its work has been done.

I popped some ice into my mouth.

"I don't want to fight my way up this climb," I declared to Rita as I rolled the frozen crystals from one cheek to the other. "I want to flow up it. So let's try this: let's try calling chemotherapy 'juice,' just like white grape juice, red cranberry juice or orange juice. Let's have ourselves a 'juice festival.' I want to imagine the juice going into me, doing its work as powerful medicine and smoothly flowing out of me. That way I can save my energy for healing."

"Sounds like a great idea," agreed Rita. "I've never heard it described that way before."

Sir Edmund Hillary once said: "Everest is never conquered. Occasionally she tolerates a momentary success." I had learned on Everest that to try to fight my way up a mountain was folly. I had to work with nature, not against her. To succeed in my cancer climb I did not want to fight chemotherapy either. We knew the strength of the chemicals Rita was giving me. That became clear as we watched the extreme care with which she handled them. The cytarabine was clear and came in a transparent plastic bag about the size of a loaf of bread. The idarubicin was red and was delivered in a prepackaged syringe. From the moment these medications arrived, Rita handled them as if they were hazardous waste. She wore blue plastic gloves to protect her hands and she never set the medications down on anything without first putting an absorbent pad underneath. The chemicals could burn the skin if spilled and the fumes they emitted were toxic. That is why they were never opened to the air, except in the pharmacist's lab under a well-ventilated hood.

So wouldn't this stuff burn its way throughout my body? Quickly, I cancelled that thought. It was precisely the mindset I wanted to avoid. I needed to think rationally and have faith in the professionals around me.

I had seen people fight their way through chemo before. Slowly, they wasted away. In the end, they did not die of cancer. They starved to death. Once they became physically weak, they became mentally weak, and once they became mentally weak, their spirits soon followed. That is what had happened to my little five-year-old nephew, Peter James. I did not want it to happen to me. Patti had warned me about taking a combative approach to cancer.

"We use words like fight, conquer, kill, battle, beat, defeat and assault in association with cancer," she had once told me. "That's how our society tells us to react – to fight for our lives, defend ourselves and compete to defeat the enemy. The problem is that this mindset creates a fight-or-flight response in us. Under these circumstances, that can be fatal.

"This isn't a war or a football match. Cancer is trillions of our own cells reproducing out of control. We can't afford to start fighting ourselves. The odds of us overcoming trillions of our own cells are less than winning the lottery.

"When we fight, adrenalin courses through our veins and we become superhumanly strong – but only for short periods of time. Coming through and recovering from illness is not a sprint. It's a climb – one that happens slowly and carefully, day after day, month after month, sometimes for years."

Now I had to put my experience and Patti's theory into practice. My life depended on it.

"If we fight," I said to Rita, "we very quickly become exhausted. But if we flow, we take on the force of a river."

> *"If we fight, we very quickly become exhausted.*
> *But if we flow, we take on the force of a river."*
>
> – Alan Hobson

After carefully ensuring my name and the patient identification number on my hospital wristband matched those on the labels affixed to the chemotherapy, Rita began to prepare the syringe of idarubicin for injection into my central line.

"Before you push that into me," I said, "could I have a moment to meditate?"

"Of course," she agreed, discreetly leaving the room.

With Cecilia sitting on my bed next to me, I disappeared within myself. I looked straight at my framed red and yellow point of pure light on the wall, the picture on which I had focused my mind hundreds of times during meditation. Then I let myself become completely calm, as if I was looking over a beautiful vista on a clear, blue-sky day.

"Baba," I prayed silently. "Please purify me with this medicine. Allow it to flow smoothly through me like juice and then gently out of me."

Then I focused only on pure white peaceful light. I imagined it emanating from above and placidly flowing through every part of my body. It made me feel warm and safe.

A minute or two passed as I hung in this blissful state. Then I slowly returned to the room.

"Are you ready?" Rita inquired, re-entering as if on cue.

"Yes," I answered.

Slowly, she attached the syringe of chemo to my central line. Then she looked at her watch.

"Idarubicin is given over ten to fifteen minutes, a little bit at a time," she explained. "During this time we carefully monitor you for potential side effects."

I breathed out, relaxing as much as I could. Rita began to push on the syringe.

I bit down on the ice in my mouth, waiting to taste something. I imagined cranberry juice flowing smoothly into my body. I tasted nothing.

"How do you feel so far?" Rita asked.

"Great," I replied.

"Wonderful," she beamed. "Let's hope that continues."

Cecilia sat beside me on the bed, holding my hand and running her fingers gently through my hair.

"You might not be able to do that much longer," I suggested.

"Maybe not," she agreed, "but I just thought I'd take advantage of the opportunity while I still had the chance."

She kissed me gently on the forehead.

The idarubicin went in without a hitch. Once it was done, Rita hoisted the bag of cytarabine up on my I.V. pole.

"Here comes the white grape juice," she announced, smiling. "If your visualization worked the first time, maybe it'll work the second time too."

Calmly, I watched the first drops of the medicine drip out of the bottom of the bag and into my line.

"How long will it take before I start to feel like I'm at high altitude?" I asked.

"It varies from patient to patient," Rita replied. "You'll probably be fine the first day, but we'll monitor you closely."

Closely she did. Every five to ten minutes at first, Rita was in my room taking my pulse, blood pressure and body temperature, and asking how I was feeling. Standard protocol required her to do this every one or two hours, but she deliberately increased the frequency just to ensure I was as comfortable as possible. She carefully noted each detail on a form at my bedside. She was methodical and absolutely meticulous. I felt safe in her care.

"You've been through this before," I remarked.

"Yes we have, Alan," she affirmed, "and we'll get through it with you too. If patients react adversely, they usually do so in the first few minutes if it's an allergic reaction or in the first few hours if it's nausea. I'm here to help you in whatever way I can."

I felt fine – so much so, in fact, that I quickly began to tire of sitting in my room, chained to an I.V. I have never been good at the waiting game. I am happiest when I am in motion. That way I feel like I am actually *doing* something. Eventually, my cancer experience would teach me otherwise – that it was possible, in fact absolutely vital, to learn that doing nothing was actually doing something. This was a huge adjustment for me.

In a few days, it would become impossible for me to stay active. Until that day came, however, I hauled myself, my pole and my bag, like a ball and chain, to the stationary bike on the ward. There, I tried to maintain a modicum of fitness, although I knew it would be fleeting.

Over the years, physical activity had become almost as much a daily part of my life as eating and sleeping. While preparing for Everest, I had developed my own training mantra. For every step I took on the treadmill, I said to myself, "CAN...WILL. I CAN climb Everest, I WILL climb Everest. I CAN climb Everest, I WILL climb Everest," over and over and over again.

On my medical mountain, I had another mantra. For every step I took on the ward while receiving chemotherapy I said to myself, "I CAN get better. I WILL get better. I CAN get better. I WILL get better." I also repeated it to myself while I was on the stationary bike on the ward. Cecilia taped a copy of this CAN/WILL mantra to the foot of my hospital bed.

After my bike session, I returned to my room. There, Cecilia and I began to develop a chemotherapy climbing plan. The first infusion was to last about a week, roughly the same amount of time it takes to climb from the base of Everest to the summit once a person is acclimatized. The closer we got to the end of the chemo cycle, the worse I was likely to feel, just like getting closer to the summit of Everest. Headaches were common. So was acute fatigue, nausea, vomiting and insomnia – precisely the same side effects chemo produced.

We tried to imagine each round of chemotherapy like a summit bid on Everest. We even posted notes on the door of my hospital room to remind us of where we were on our climb.

Our first note said, "August 12. Day 1. Base Camp," our second, "August 13. Day 2. Camp 1," our third, "August 14. Day 3. Camp 2" and so on up the peak.

Chemo could take me part way up my medical mountain. If it could put my leukemia into remission and if an adult blood stem cell or bone marrow match could be found, a transplant might take me a giant leap closer to a return to full health. Of course the unknowns would not end there. I would still have to build myself back to full fitness after the transplant and no one seemed to have any idea how long that might take or even if it was possible. The best scenario, from diagnosis through treatment, transplant and recovery would take three to five years to complete – about the same amount of time it took to put together a typical Everest expedition.

The simple act of taking charge by making a plan somehow seemed to make all the unknowns less intimidating. Linking my present situation with a successful experience I had had in the past helped considerably. It transformed the unknown into the known. Now all we had to do was execute our plan.

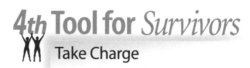

4th Tool for *Survivors*
Take Charge

Providentially, a Sherpa appeared to help get us focused. My best friend, Dale Ens, arrived for his first visit.

Dale stood about 5 foot 8, and was wiry and fit. His deep-set dark eyes, thin lips and bushy eyebrows were complemented by an equally thick moustache. The skin on his face was drawn back tightly against his high cheek bones, and although he was not gaunt, he always reminded me of Shakespeare's characterization of Cassius in the famous drama *Julius Caesar* – he had "a lean and hungry look."

I had known Dale since moving to Calgary fifteen years earlier. We had met at a local swimming pool where he had been training for triathlons. He was an intense but fun-loving man with a charismatic personality. His razor-sharp wit and bone-dry sense of humor made him a stimulating and entertaining conversationalist and an impressive orator. He could always be relied upon for rapid repartee and clever comebacks, but he was also fiercely reasoned and analytical. He made his living as one of the city's best estate planners, and he could swiftly dissect even the most complex financial and life insurance cases. He was always honest, often painfully frank, but also highly perceptive and insightful. Since the birth of his only daughter, Georgia, seven years earlier, his softer side had come forward and helped to mold him into a wise and well-rounded man of considerable depth and kindness. It was this rare combination of wit, wisdom and benevolence that I loved so much about him. You could trust him with your life, especially in a crisis.

Dale cruised into my room spouting his usual sarcasm.

"Hobson," he said brashly. "You've really done it this time. As if Everest wasn't enough, you've landed your butt in a hospital bed, and now Cecilia and I are going to have to bail you out. You could at least have given us some advance notice. This is completely unacceptable."

Then he looked at me with grave concern and gave me a huge, long hug. Tears welled up in his eyes.

"This is not good, pal," he said, changing his tone completely and motioning to my I.V. unit. "If you think you can get that tree you're tied to uprooted, we need to talk. Can you walk?"

"Absolutely," I said, swinging out of bed.

Dale rallies to the defense of his friends like no one else I have ever known. Years before, his friend and business partner, Bill McDonald, had been critically injured while Dale and Bill were on a motorcycle trip in Idaho. Dale had almost single-handedly coordinated the rescue effort and Bill's initial medical treatment, and had stayed in close contact during the years of convalescence that followed. During that time, he had handled almost all of Bill's financial affairs, coordinated his insurance coverage and exercised power of attorney.

We walked to the elevator and rode down to the ground floor.

"This sucks," he grumbled as we entered the hospital lobby. "This really sucks, Al."

"Yeah, Dale," I agreed, "I guess it does. But what the hell are you supposed to do? Crying isn't going to help a damn. Self-pity doesn't work either. Neither does trying to figure out how this could have possibly happened in the first place. If I knew that, I'd be up for the Nobel Prize for Medicine. As it is, the only prize I'm going to get today is this big bag of grape juice and maybe a chance at a longer life. I'm just going to have to take my medicine and hope for the best."

"True, Hobson, but this is really tough medicine," he bemoaned. "This is the kind of medicine that can kill you."

"So can no medicine at all and quite frankly, given the alternative, I'd rather go down trying than just roll over and play dead."

There was a long pause.

"Okay," he relented, "so there's not a damn thing we can do about it. If that's the case, which it is, then here's what we're going to do…"

Over the next five minutes, Dale laid out a six-month plan for my life. He explained that with my power of attorney, he and Cecilia would take care of my business, bills, will, medical directives and all my financial affairs.

"You only need to concentrate on one thing," he counseled, "– getting better. For the next six months, that's where I want you to put your entire focus. We'll take care of the rest."

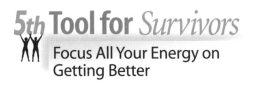

5th Tool for *Survivors*
Focus All Your Energy on Getting Better

"Thank you so much," I said, choking back the tears. "You are a good man, Ensy, the best. I am so lucky to have you in my life."

"Luck has nothing to do with it," he countered, reverting once again to his caustic charm. "I can no more rid my life of your shining face than I can rid myself of gum on the bottom of my shoe. We're stuck together, you and I, and we'll probably stay that way for the rest of your life…"

Then he realized what he had said.

"I can only hope that the rest of your life is a very long time," he insisted as the tears started to run down his cheeks. We wept together.

"Why is it that you seem to end up in these roles?" I asked when we had both dried our eyes. "I mean, you were there for Bill and voilà, history repeats itself only a few years later with me."

"I don't know, Al," he reflected. "And you know what? It doesn't matter. None of that means anything right now. What matters is that you get the best medical care possible, the best support your friends can give you, and that you get back on your feet and out of this place just as soon as you possibly can. I love you and I believe in you. You can do it."

Success is…the caring shoulder of a friend. It's knowing we're not alone, feeling we belong and knowing that somehow, somewhere, someone cares. Amid the chaos of change around us, there is someone waiting for us at the bottom of the slope.

– The Triumph of Tenacity
(formerly titled, The Power of Passion)

CHAPTER 6

Cecilia
DEJA
VU

A few days ago, I didn't know the Foothills Hospital existed. Now I spend more time here than at our apartment.

I am restless, and the pale yellow walls of Alan's hospital room close in on me. The window is my only escape from the dreariness of the cancer ward. I know that Alan has a more upbeat view of our surroundings, but I don't feel that way. I have done my best to create a warm environment in this sterile world in which we now find ourselves. No fragrant lilacs here, no warm breezes – only disinfectant scents the stale air of Unit 57. I have decorated the room with photographs of our friends and family, and brought in placemats and silverware for when we eat. But nothing can change the fact that we are confined to a hospital room with oxygen bottles on the walls and signs warning visitors to wash their hands.

I need to move. I want to go for a run, but I settle for a walk around the ward. It is the first of several nights I will venture from the confines of our eight-by-ten foot hospital room. I look over at Alan to see that he is resting comfortably and let him know I need to take a walk. I get up from the stiff vinyl chair and give him a kiss, whispering that I'll be back soon to say goodnight.

It is nearly 11 p.m., and the unappetizing odors of the institutional evening meals still linger in the hall. The incessant intercom calls out nurses' names, names I am coming to know well. They echo through my head as I walk.

I step softly so I won't disturb the other patients. Most have their doors closed to stop the irritating fluorescent hall lights from keeping them awake, although night is not a time for rest here. While much of the activity slows down, it never stops. There are continual interruptions for blood pressure, temperature readings and medication. I have learned that I have to go home and sleep in my own bed, or at least rest in my own bed at night. Sleep deprivation takes its toll. I cannot afford to become sick, so I go home each night, eventually.

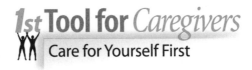

1st Tool for *Caregivers*
Care for Yourself First

The nurses' station is quiet at this hour. The nurses have completed their reports and the night shift has replaced the afternoon. The ward takes on a somber feel. As I near the station, I see a blonde woman in her mid-forties dressed in comfortable pants and a loose top sitting with a nurse. One thing you learn very quickly is to wear comfortable clothes. This is a place where you sit most of your day and night away. Comfort is essential.

The nurse glances up at me. I guess I have been staring at the two of them. I am astonished by what I see. I look at this forty-something woman and see myself when I was sixteen. She must have just received the prognosis for her mother.

I flash back to Hotel Dieu Hospital in the summer of 1974 in New Orleans. My mother is in for surgery, a double mastectomy, to remove the cancer from her body. My father and my aunt are in the waiting room with me. When the doctor walks into the room, everyone knows the news is not good. He says the cancer has spread throughout her body. There isn't anything else he can do. She has six months to a year to live.

I am an only child, so I take on many of the household responsibilities. The word cancer, the chemotherapy and radiation treatments and their side effects are not discussed openly. Much of the time I am reeling with self-doubt. How can I help my mother through this? I do what I can. Throughout it all, my mother never complains, never stops and never gives up.

One day I come home from an outing with a friend to find my mother unconscious on the living room floor. I call an ambulance but my mother dies en route to the hospital. I still carry the guilt and self-blame for not being there with her during her last moments on Earth. Thankfully, I also carry some of her strength.

The blonde woman on Unit 57 is sobbing uncontrollably. Why is this woman crying? Her mother isn't dead. She still has time to say, "I love you." She hasn't been deprived of their time together. She's had more than forty years with her mother. What does she have to cry about? If only I'd had time to grieve before my mother abandoned me.

I feel violated that this woman's grief is spreading through the ward, that this expression of emotion is taking place. I don't want to see this. I can't sympathize with her, I can't cry with her. I don't want to cry with her. I turn away, avoiding eye contact. The nurse holds the woman to her chest.

This is all a bad dream. I'm not here on Unit 57 caring for Alan. I'm not among dying patients. I want to run out, but all I can do is turn and walk back to Alan's room. There, I can recover. There, I can see him still healthy. The chemo treatments have not yet taken their toll – oh, but they will. I know what's coming and it won't be pretty.

Stop it, stop the negative thoughts right now. Turn away from the pain, from the dying. Turn to the strong.

Strength is my only salvation. I will be strong and positive. Just because my past experience was not the outcome I would have liked doesn't mean this outcome will be the same. It is too early to tell. Don't go there. Don't allow the pain to destroy hope.

CHAPTER 7

Alan

THE CLIMB
BEGINS

"If you want to master your situation, control your fear."

– Mr. Laurie Skreslet,
First Canadian to Climb Mt. Everest,
One Step Beyond

…After surviving the night alone in base camp with only a mild headache that soon went away, I decided to reconnoiter the route…My plan ran into its first snag when I couldn't eat breakfast because I was nauseous from the altitude. All I could manage to hold down was half a quart of sugar-free apple cider. I have no idea why we purchased sugar-free mixes for our trip. As one of the biggest single struggles we have on Everest is keeping our weight loss to an absolute minimum, it was ludicrous to have diet drinks along. I laughed when I read the package.

For another high altitude climber, climbing on no breakfast might not have been so bad, but my metabolism must have food, especially when I am working hard. If there's no fuel for my fire, I very quickly burn out.

This is what happened to me the first time I tried to ascend…I was reduced to a snail's pace as I struggled to will out every step. I felt like I was an actor in some kind of bad slow-motion movie. It took so much effort just to take a single step. I reminded myself that it would probably be even tougher higher up, so I tried to view this experience as a learning opportunity – a chance to further harden myself for the hardships that were to come. The primary challenge of Everest is fought within ourselves, where all of our battles are won or lost in life.

– From Everest to Enlightenment

Rolling over too many times in the same direction is not a good idea when you are tied to an I.V. The second night in the hospital, I awoke at 3 a.m. desperately needing the bathroom, but so entangled in my I.V. line I could not move my hands. In the dark, in a place still unfamiliar to me, I wondered how I was going to make it to the toilet in time. Meanwhile, the alarm on my I.V. pump was sounding to indicate a blocked line, but I could not free my hands even to reach the nurse call button.

After a lot of frantic flailing, I managed to extricate myself just in time to make it to the toilet. When I returned to my bed, a young nurse appeared to take my nightly blood sample. She began to peer inquisitively at my central line. I knew I was in trouble when she queried, "Do you happen to know which one of these I'm supposed to use?"

"Which one of what?" I asked.

"*These!*" she indicated, showing me the three separate needle ports coming off my central line.

"Looks like you've got a one-in-three chance," I braved. "They all seem to be coming from the same place, so I'd say you should probably be okay with any one of them."

That was not good enough for her. She decided to wait until 7 a.m. for the day nurse. Then she left and I was alone with my thoughts.

How the hell did I end up in here? What was I doing in a hospital bed? Was this some kind of crazy dream?

I tossed and turned, struggling with my cursed I.V. line. I wanted to yank it from my chest, trash the pump to pieces and storm off the ward.

Anger is not a good thing when you are trying to fall asleep. It creates adrenalin and adrenalin creates energy. I finally fell asleep around 5 a.m. and had only two short hours of uncomfortable respite before the day nurse woke me to take the missed blood sample.

Getting adequate rest in a hospital, as any patient knows, is next to impossible, especially on an acute care ward. At night you are awakened every three or four hours so the staff can reassure themselves you are still breathing. Charting your pulse and blood pressure seems to take precedence over everything else.

During the day it is no different. It is impossible to rest. You are interrupted every few minutes by announcements over the ward intercom, or by doctors, nurses, visitors, lab technicians, porters, cleaners, counselors, dieticians, physiotherapists, pharmacists and so on. While I appreciated this impressive level of care, there was no way I could have adequate rest for my body to heal.

Sleep deprivation now added to the trials of my medical mountain and reminded me again of life at high altitude. Stricken with nausea, headaches and exhaustion from life in the rarefied air, climbers quickly become physically and emotionally drained. Despite this, it is sometimes impossible to doze off because the body's delicate sleep mechanism is completely disrupted. Even if you are fortunate enough to fall asleep at night, you frequently awaken a short while later, frightened to death in the darkness of your tent, alone and gasping for air. This can go on for weeks during an expedition. Each day you get progressively weaker. Finally, summit day arrives, the day when you need to be at your strongest, and you are actually at your weakest. This expedition was already starting to seem comparable.

Within days of being admitted to the hospital, I realized it was essential that I escape from the debilitating routine. I looked at the pigeons amassing on the ledge outside my window. I envied them. They could fly wherever they chose and sleep whenever they wanted. I wanted to taste that kind of freedom again, but now that possibility seemed unattainably distant. I imagined myself pecking at the pane like a pigeon behind glass, but it was like a quarter-inch mile. I hoped beyond hope that some day the window would crack and I could make my way to freedom in the great wide world on the other side. For every minute I spent inside the glass, I wanted a thousand more outside it in the future.

I remembered the words of Jacob Riis, the American photographer, journalist and author: "When nothing seems to help, I go and look at the stonecutter hammering away at his rock perhaps a hundred times without as much as a crack showing in it. Yet at the hundred and first blow, it will split in two, and I know it was not that blow that did it – but all that had gone before."

I vowed to keep chipping away at life. As I lay in bed that night, a powerful vision began to play on the screen of my mind. I remembered the yawning ice crevasses I had faced as a mountaineer: those huge cracks in glaciers, some hundreds of feet deep and many hundreds of feet wide, twisted, sometimes sinister looking and always dangerous. If they are narrow, the force of the wind can fill in the gap across their mouths with snow, making them invisible from above. But just inches below the surface, they can widen into massive crystalline caverns that can swallow a house. If you fall into one without the proper safety equipment and training and without a partner, you will likely never come out. You die of exposure or from the injuries sustained when you plunge into the depths.

I had tumbled into just such a deadly crevasse, the crevasse of cancer. It could swallow my body, shatter my spirit and take my life.

This terrifying realization forced me to re-evaluate my life. The urgency of recent events had galvanized in my mind what I instinctively knew in my heart and in my soul – that I was not ready to die. I had been incredibly fortunate to get safely up and down Everest, but I did not want my legacy to be that I had climbed a mountain. I wanted more – more dreams, more adventures and most importantly, more meaning. I wanted to inspire others and make a difference. I had achieved one of my dreams, but now I wanted to help others achieve theirs. There were more important mountains to climb. I had to get out of here and back on those peaks. Somehow, I had to climb back.

As my eyelids drooped after the 7 a.m. blood drawing and I began to doze back to sleep, someone entered my room – singing. Opening my eyes wider, I was surprised to see a small, dark-haired man smoothly sweeping a mop under my bed.

"Good morning," I mumbled, struggling to bring the day into focus.

"Good morning, sir," he replied cheerfully. "I am so sorry to wake you. I'll just be a moment."

Niceto "Ceto" Gile, I learned, was a Filipino Canadian. A father of two, he worked two jobs seven days a week, three hundred sixty-five days a year to support his young family. His other job was as a caretaker at the University of Calgary. Yet despite his heavy workload, he was positively radiant. His face glowed and he sang the entire time he was in my room. Within minutes, he was finished. He bid me a pleasant goodbye and left the room. Every time I saw him for months afterwards, he was exactly the same. He became a sort of talisman, one of the earliest members of my newly forming team.

After he left, I stared up at my I.V. pole.

"There must be some way to get that thing into a backpack so I can carry it around," I thought. My mind began to spin with ideas.

That is when Rita arrived.

"Good morning, Alan," she chirped in her usual sweet way. "How was your night?"

"A bit rough," I lamented. "I'm having a hard time getting used to hospital time. I found myself reliving the movie *Born Free*. I lay awake trying to figure out how to dismantle this I.V. pump and put it into a backpack. Do you think anyone would object if I took it apart?"

"Before you do that," she said diplomatically, "let me go and make a few inquiries and see what can be done."

She was back a short while later with the ward nurse, who to my amazement was carrying a small I.V. pump and waist pack.

I jumped up and down like a little boy at a party. As soon as they had me hooked up to the pump, I bolted from the room and headed straight for the stairs. Before I got there, the door to the stairwell opened and Cecilia appeared. She gave me a great big hug and a kiss and declared, "My heavens! It sure didn't take you long to get loose. We're going to have to figure out some other way to get you to stay in bed."

"Quick," I implored, "let's get out of here."

"Soon," she replied with restraint. "First, let's make sure you have some breakfast. Where you're headed, you're going to need every calorie we can get into you."

When we returned to my room, Bolek, a personal care assistant, was waiting to take my weight. I stepped on the scale.

"It might be a good idea if you take off that waist pack," he said chuckling. "A bag of chemo weighs over two pounds and I don't want the doctors to think you're drinking it. I haven't seen a patient yet who naturally gained weight during treatment, but maybe you could be the first."

Bolek Babiarz was another gem like Rita. A Polish immigrant who had fled the communist occupation with his wife and son years before, he had since devoted his life to brightening the lives of others on Unit 57. In the process he had earned a reputation for compassion, kindness and especially creativity. My personalized wall calendar, on which the nurses logged my daily blood cell counts, had been hand painted by him. Every patient admitted to the ward received one as Bolek's personal gift.

Bolek was composed, soft-spoken and somewhat shy, but his kind and gentle exterior concealed a fiercely competitive drive. A former nationally ranked professional soccer player in his native Poland, he stood well over six feet, and although he was not as physically fit as he had once been, he carried himself with strength and presence. He had soft facial features, a high forehead and a receding hairline, and his full, round face was tinged with a perpetual five o'clock shadow. Wherever he went on the ward, two things always went with him – his blue hospital fatigues and his grey, V-necked vest sweater. It said much about the man – that he was willing to roll up his shirtsleeves and do the dirty work if necessary, but he was also warm-hearted. He spoke with a thick accent, but his sympathetic eyes and smile communicated beyond words. They said he was your friend.

The scale showed I weighed one hundred fifty-one pounds. I knew from previous experience that I had less than ten pounds of fat to lose before I would start losing precious muscle and strength. My weight became a vital measure of my health, and Cecilia and I watched it diligently. We knew that if it fell below one hundred forty-five pounds, things might start to get scary. There was a direct relationship between weight and life.

Cecilia went to the door and posted the day's note:

"Aug. 13. Day 2. Camp 1, 19,200 feet."

Rita returned to my room. She gave me my second dose of idarubicin "cranberry juice" and ensured my cytarabine "grape juice" was still running smoothly. I could already feel myself heading downhill. It registered in an increasing nausea, mild headache and a general feeling of lassitude. I tried a few minutes of physical activity on the stationary bike, but it was pointless. I just did not have it in me.

By now, word had spread among my friends and colleagues that I was in hospital. For the next few days, I received a steady stream of visitors. I was deeply touched to see them, but I soon learned that as the chemo took effect, my energy level declined. This, unfortunately, made it increasingly difficult for me to see many visitors. If I hoped to regain my health, I had to conserve my energy, even with my friends.

One of the visitors that day was my meditation instructor, Valerie Simonson. We had met shortly after my last Everest expedition. From the first time we spoke, I sensed something special about her. It emanated from her peaceful face, frequent laughter and bubbly personality. She is a strikingly tall, blue-eyed woman with shoulder-length blonde hair and a vibrant personality. She teaches open eye meditation and is a yogi.

Valerie had given up a successful corporate career to seek a deeper purpose in life and she had found it in Raja Yoga. Only after gaining a new spiritual perspective and adopting a devout lifestyle had she eventually returned to work as an investment consultant. She was an enigma – a deeply spiritual person and an entrepreneur.

"*Raja* means 'king' and yoga means 'connection,'" she explained during my first lesson. "If happiness is a state of mind, then we need to learn to rule our state. Raja Yoga helps us do just that."

The concept of being king over one's thoughts immediately intrigued me. If I could learn to do that, I might also learn how to manage my emotions. Rather than react instinctively to life's situations and become overwhelmed by fear and other negative feelings, I might be able to seize control. Even if only a fraction of what she was offering was attainable, the benefits could be immeasurable. As the Roman philosopher, Lucius Seneca, once said, "Most powerful is he who has himself in his power."

"You are about to test the power of Raja Yoga to its fullest," Valerie predicted calmly as she sat beside me on my bed. "Amidst your fear and uncertainty, you must find peace."

Carefully, Valerie opened a small package she had brought with her. In it was a tiny, oval-shaped red pin with an imitation diamond in the middle of it. I knew from her teachings as a member of the Brahma Kumaris, or "B.K.s," of India, that this "stone" was believed to be a representation of a human soul shining brightly as a point of light.

What separates the B.K.s from many other spiritual followers I have discovered in my travels is that they accept and, indeed, embrace all spiritual paths and all people. There are some six thousand centers of The Brahma Kumaris World Spiritual University worldwide with millions of students and teachers involved in classes in eighty-six countries. Some of their leading yogis have advised the United Nations on how to make the world a more harmonious, productive and peaceful place. Human beings, the B.K.s assert, are souls contained in bodies and each person has a role to play in the human drama of the corporeal world, even terrorists, dictators and other villains. Thus no matter what an individual's role, gender, age, nationality, race, economic status or religion, they are all souls. The pure simplicity of this appealed to my sense of practicality. It worked –

anywhere, with anyone, at any time.

During my illness, many B.K.s would visit us. All of them came, as my family and friends did, with an open heart and sincere wishes. To us, it did not really matter where they derived their sense of compassion – only that they had it and took the time to share it with us. For this, we will be eternally grateful. Through Valerie and other spiritual mentors, we have come to realize that family can go far beyond blood relations. The day she came to visit, I received a gift I might never have received were it not for cancer – I gained a sister.

Cradling the pin in her palm, Valerie looked straight into my eyes.

"You have now embarked on a great voyage of discovery and adventure," she imparted. "In your journey you will meet many. You will know to whom to give this next."

Then she hugged me and left the room.

I had grown up in a rough-and-tumble household of four boys where spirituality was all but absent. My father was a research scientist who worked for Canada's National Research Council for thirty-two years. He had three university degrees, including a Ph.D. in physics, and had helped develop the instruments used to measure the atmospheric pressure on the moon during the Apollo 12, 14 and 15 missions. He believed that if something did not register on a gauge, it did not exist. He admitted to the presence of the invisible atom and other sub-atomic particles only because of the irrefutable scientific evidence they existed. At home, we did not worship, we did not read religious texts, and we rarely said grace before meals. As far as my father was concerned, there was no such thing as a Higher Power and the mere suggestion He might exist caused him to bristle.

"Prove it!" he would say defiantly. Spirituality as a subject, at least until much later in his life, was taboo.

My experiences on Everest and with cancer would challenge the deep-seated belief system my father had instilled in me as a child. In the mountains, I had realized there was a natural, almost mystical balance of action and reaction, yin and yang, just as there was night and day, freezing and thawing. It is impossible to be on Everest and not feel the presence of a Higher Power. That Power is as obvious as the awesome size of Everest herself. It makes a definitive impression beyond words. Sometimes, the only sound It makes is in the sound of the raging wind. At other times, the mountain is so silent you can hear It. In this world of extremes, I discovered my own spirituality.

It was this inner voice that spoke to me often on 57 and during the rest of our cancer journey. It said that my life's song was not over and that I deeply wanted to keep singing it. Whether I would get that opportunity or not was still unclear.

I had never been on a mountain this intangible before. I knew there was a summit somewhere, but I sure could not see it. I had no idea how I was going to get there, or even if I could. It was like climbing blind. I knew I could plummet to my death at any moment, but I just had to keep climbing. Such was life on "Mt. Nebulous."

Now, only two days into the expedition, our support team was taking shape. As the chemo started to work, my nausea increased and my motivation decreased. But even as my inner world was shrinking, my outer circle of support was expanding far beyond the hospital. Around me, the Sherpas were starting to assemble. As they did, I could feel a load lifting from my shoulders. One by one, each of them picked up a portion of my burden and headed up the hill ahead of me. I was buoyed by a force larger than Everest. I could not touch it, I could not see it, but it was there.

Our expedition was underway.

CHAPTER 8

Cecilia
SUPPORT FROM ALL SIDES

Every health professional who enters Alan's hospital room is another source of information. I hang on their every word. I write it all down. My hand is in motion like a sewing machine's needle, stitching together the patchwork of information. The pattern is not clear to me, but I continue to take notes anyway. I know I must learn as much as possible about Alan's condition. This time around, unlike with my mother, I will have the information to be a better caregiver. Taking notes is my first line of defense.

I do the same thing at home. Feverishly, I pore through websites for statistics in our favor. Hours pass, but it seems that all I can find are negative stats. My heart aches for just one case study with a better than fifty percent chance of survival. Pieces of paper are spread all over the living room floor like pieces of a jigsaw puzzle. I try to formulate a picture in my mind but there are too many missing pieces. The picture is clouded in fear. The more I read, the more fearful I become.

I will have to contain my fear. I will have to let go of my past experience with cancer. We have everything in our favor. Alan is tough and ready. We have the best medical care. I cannot allow myself to become lost in the negative numbers. I will remain calm, I will remain positive, I will move past my fear into freedom.

2nd Tool for *Caregivers*
Put Your Fears Aside

I am grateful that Alan receives so many visitors, although in some ways it's a mixed blessing. He takes the time with each one to explain how the leukemic cells have overrun his blood stream. Our friends listen intently. Their faces express concern and compassion. I log each visit in my journal and decorate the walls of the hospital room with their get-well cards.

As dusk falls over the city and the room takes on the unnatural glow of the fluorescent lights, I look over at Alan to see fatigue in his face. The chemo is taking its toll. I have seen this look before and realize we must conserve his energy. He knows the key to a successful climb lies in the prudent allocation of his own resources. We both agree that I will take on the difficult task of managing visitors. This is totally against my southern roots, but it is essential to Alan's health and that is all that matters.

I pull out my pen and journal, sit down in the recliner next to his bed and proceed to make a list of dos and don'ts. I entitle it, "How to Be Alan's Best Climbing Partner."

#1: Call before coming. If our friends call first, I will have an opportunity to let them know if Alan's energy reserves are full – or fully depleted. This way I will not be in the awkward position of turning them away once they have taken the time and made the effort to come to the hospital.

#2: No hugs please – warm handshakes only. Outwardly, Alan's chest may appear normal, but underneath his T-shirt, the incision made for his central line is still tender. With every hug, I watch him grimace.

#3: Limit visits to twenty minutes. With keen interest, Alan catches up with his friends' daily lives. I observe as he asks probing questions. Then I see his eyelids begin to drop and I know it's time to conclude the visit. This is always a hard thing for me to do.

#4: No visitors after 8 p.m. By 8 p.m., Alan's energy is close to gone.

#5: One visitor at a time. Alan is a sensitive man. He speaks to the uniqueness of each one in the room. This takes concentration. Chemotherapy zaps his mental resources. As Alan rises to the test of speaking to each person, his energy slips further down the slope.

#6: Cheerful smiles and laughter only. We find smiles and laughter recharge our batteries, while sadness drains them. All of our friends and family embrace this idea.

I post the note on the door to Alan's room. Later, I notice people reading it. I had been concerned that others might find it offensive, but everyone seems completely understanding and supportive.

We are grateful for our climbing team. Together, we are stronger.

CHAPTER 9

Alan

CAMP 1

"Your moment of greatest strength is your moment of greatest singleness of purpose."

– Mr. Laurie Skreslet,
First Canadian to Climb Mt. Everest,
One Step Beyond

I have never gotten used to the early rises so frequent in climbing. We call them "alpine starts," but for me…they don't start fast.

When you wake up in your own bed at home all you have to do is roll out of it in your pj's, strip to the buff, step into the nice hot shower and voilà, you enter the world warmly.

At high altitude, when you wake up in the morning, you enter the world abruptly. The first thing that hits you is the freezing cold air. It strikes you like a slap in the face, welcoming you suddenly to your new reality. Your first reaction is to dive back into your bag and try to come to your senses.

To get out of your sleeping bag without freezing, you have to get dressed in your bag before you actually get out of it. This is akin to putting on all your clothes, including your winter jacket, hat, scarf and gloves, before you pull back the sheets. The last thing you want to do is get out of your bag buck-naked. That would definitely be a rude awakening – one even ruder than rising at 4 a.m.

– From Everest to Enlightenment

Most patients die at night. It is a harsh truth that when we are left alone in the dark, our thoughts can be very poor company. The medical system has thus adopted cycles to check in with patients every few hours during the night. This means sleep deprivation has become a way of life. On Unit 57, there was an almost pathological need among the nurses to ensure no one died on *their* shift, even though, of course, that was impossible. This guard dog mentality pervaded the whole staff. Nurses with decades of experience, who had seen death many times, tried to stave off the moment of passing, if not for the patient, then for their loved ones. While everyone understood that that decision was not in their hands, the staff still hoped to influence the outcome, even if death could ultimately be a gift.

This constantly shifting landscape between life and death made 57 an enigmatic place. Everyone knew the possibility of death was present, but no one except perhaps the terminally ill patients was going to allow it to rear its head if they had any say in the matter. This was not a desire among the staff to prolong life unnecessarily. It was their desire to perform at their peak so that in the end, whatever the outcome, there would be no dishonor. I liked that about 57. There was a truthfulness to the place that reminded me of the mountains. It was as if cancer, like a mountain, stripped away the thin superficial veneer that sometimes covers our lives and revealed the core of what really mattered underneath. Life on the edge was like a steep mountain ridge – although sometimes obscured in cloud, the edge was always there, sharp, exposed and brutally honest. If the staff missed a detail or made a mistake, someone could die. Vigilance was vital.

On my third afternoon, I was told to report for a "MUGA scan." As I had no idea what that was and no one seemed able to tell me, I immediately became fearful. My mind quickly raced toward ruin. *Were they searching for more cancer? Did I have undetected tumors? What was going on?*

We soon tracked down Dr. Shane Devlin, the resident on the ward. He was the most junior physician, but he made the majority of the routine day-to-day medical decisions. He worked brutally long hours, functioned on only a few hours sleep and seemed to walk the ridge almost as closely as some of the patients.

In spite of his fatigue and crushing load, Shane greeted me with a smile. He was clearly tired, but if he was stressed, he did not seem to show it. In a remarkable display of lucidity, he was quick to read my apprehension and even quicker to address it.

"A MUGA? Stands for Multi-Gated Acquisition scan," he explained. "Routine stuff, Al. It's just a standard test we do with first round chemo patients to ensure your heart is pumping properly. Some of the chemo can be hard on the heart, so before too much of it hits your system, we want to see where you're starting from. Not to worry. You'll be just fine."

At 3 p.m., the porter arrived to take me to the test. He insisted I go in a wheelchair, saying I might need it after the procedure. I was adamantly against it – I was working to maintain my independence, and I would sooner die than sit in a wheelchair until such time as I was unable to walk on my own. I had also decided not to wear the hospital clothing provided to me. This served to create a psychological separation between myself and the institution and reduced, at least in my mind, the width of the crevasse we had to cross. As I saw it, the more institutionalized I allowed myself to become, the more I had surrendered to the disease and allowed myself to become truly "hospitalized." If I was going to be a survivor, I had to start acting like one. I had to think it, say it and live it.

I started by calling myself a survivor. Medically, I was classified as a patient, but I was still alive, and in my mind this fact made me a cancer survivor. So, that is what I called myself and everything I did was aimed at maximizing the chances of staying that way. I was not a statistic. I was not a "leukemic." I was a survivor. Period.

Fortunately, the staff of 57 never once confronted me on these attitudes and behaviors, at least as long as I remained "healthy." I knew, however, that if my weight dropped and my spirits flagged, my resistance to conformity and regimentation would likely not be tolerated. So far, I appeared to be weathering my first experience with chemo reasonably well. My spirits remained relatively high, and physically I was still strong. The porter wisely sensed it might be better not to press the issue and we both left on foot.

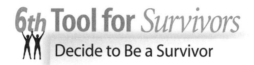

6th Tool for *Survivors*
Decide to Be a Survivor

Minutes later, we arrived at the Nuclear Medicine Department. Like most of the radiological procedure rooms, it was in the basement of the hospital. The place seemed dark and confining, but it did not stay that way for long. We soon met Peter Porcellato, a sneaker-shod nuclear medicine technologist whose laid-back, easygoing demeanor, soft speech and unpretentious manner quickly reassured me.

"Have a seat right over here, Alan," he said, motioning me toward a small cubicle. "Have you ever been 'MUGAed' before?"

"No, is this a criminal matter? If it is, I'm outta here right now and you, Peter, you're in a whole mess of trouble."

"No need to call the cops," he said, smiling broadly. Then he explained the procedure. "What I'll do is tag your blood with a radioisotope and then I'll send you into radiology so they can take a few pictures of your heart."

Sounded simple enough. The problem was that to perform the scan he would have to insert a foot-long catheter into my arm and leave it there for about twenty minutes.

By now, I was really starting to feel the effects of the chemo. I was light-headed, slightly nauseous and weak. Minutes after the catheter was inserted, I started to feel sick to my stomach.

"It's basin time again," I grimaced.

Cecilia produced one and I did my thing. Soon after that, I could feel the blood draining from my head.

"I think I'm going to pass out," I declared mechanically.

Peter moved swiftly. He removed the mattress from a nearby gurney and placed it on the floor at my feet. Then he and Cecilia slowly lifted me from my cubicle and lowered me carefully onto the mat.

"I'm losing my hearing," I said as the lights started to go out. "Counting down from five, four, three…"

I made it to the mat not a moment too soon. Somehow I maintained a vague consciousness and even kept my catheter in place.

"Thank you for that, Peter," I breathed when I began to feel a little clearer a few minutes later. "This is obviously not the first time this has happened."

"No, Alan, it isn't, but I'm glad to see you're feeling better."

"How do you stay so calm?" I asked.

"If you don't have compassion," he responded, "you have no business working here."

This and other small but affecting displays of humanity gradually altered the way I perceived the hospital. I never enjoyed being there, but when I was in need, someone capable always materialized to help. Quality, I knew, was never an accident. I wondered who was running the place. Whoever it was, was doing a fine job.

Cecilia and I made it back to the room without the need of a porter or a wheelchair. But no sooner had I arrived than I began to throw up again.

"When was the last time you took a Zofran?" Cecilia asked.

"A little over eight hours ago," I replied.

"A *little* over?" she exclaimed. "How much over?"

I was in no condition to answer.

At that moment, my brother Eric arrived for a visit. He was the picture of a seasoned businessman, his six foot frame clad in a well-pressed suit and tie, fine black leather shoes and matching socks. His full face sported a neatly clipped salt-and-pepper beard and a wide smile that lit up the room. He was his usual self – vigorous and comical.

"Looks like it's another day at the office," he remarked in his deep voice.

"Just think, I gave up a dull board meeting for this."

"Sorry about that," I said, embarrassed. "But it kinda goes with the territory."

Eric was forty-six, four years my senior. He had had a very successful series of careers as an electrical engineer, a marketer of crude oil and a telecommunications tycoon. Now he was one of the lead players in a start-up interactive media entertainment company. I love Eric very much. Despite his considerable professional success, he is still the brother I knew as a boy. He is fun and flamboyant and has the amazing ability to add a touch of levity to any situation, no matter how emotionally charged. Although a highly intelligent and sophisticated entrepreneur, he carries no airs and this perhaps as much as anything has been one of the keys to his success. His greatest passions in life are fishing, business, family and friends, probably in that order. In stark contrast with myself, he is easygoing and exceptionally witty. His light unpretentious exterior masks a passionate ambition and considerable life experience. You can always count on him for sage advice.

"Just as advertised," Eric commented, putting his hand gently on my shoulder. "This too will pass – like bad gas."

My day nurse soon appeared. "How did the test go?" she inquired.

"It was a bit of an adventure," I reported. "I've been struggling ever since."

"So I hear," she responded, nodding knowingly. "We'll just watch you for a few more minutes and see how you do. It might have nothing to do with the MUGA scan. It could simply be that your Zofran has run out."

After a few minutes of shaking heaves, it seemed obvious it had. So she swiftly hoisted a bag of the medication onto my I.V. pole and infused the anti-nauseant through the second of the ports on my central line. Within minutes, the eruptions stopped.

"That stuff is magic," I declared.

"Seems that way," Cecilia agreed, "but obviously only if we keep to the schedule. From now on, we're not going to wait eight hours for symptoms to appear. We're going to keep you medicated every seven and a half hours, day and night."

As visiting hours drew to a close and Eric prepared to leave, one of the nurses came by to announce a late visitor. My heart skipped a beat when I heard who it was. He bounced crisply into the room, fit and tanned, his angular features exuding life and energy. Just under six feet tall with a full head of long uncombed blond hair that hung down over penetrating brown eyes, Laurie Skreslet was the epitome of a rugged mountaineer. The skin on his face had been hardened by years of exposure to the sun, wind and cold, and his fingers were thick and ropey. You could tell they had spent years being jammed into rock cracks because they were spotted with scars. His nose was sharply defined, much like the ice tools he used to chop his way up severely exposed ice and snow faces in the dead of winter. On the side of his right cheek was a small but noticeable mole he had had for years. It was the lone irregularity in a face of distinct determination. His voice was deep and authoritative, his aura intense. In decades of climbing, he had pioneered first ascents of some of the most difficult and remote frozen waterfalls in the Canadian Rockies. But his most public accomplishment was being the first Canadian to climb Everest.

My relationship with Laurie went back almost twenty years to 1982 when I had offered to write his biography. The story of his Everest expedition was transfixing. His group was the first Canada had sent to the mountain, but early on, four climbers died and half of the team left Nepal amid a storm of accusations and acrimony. The expedition was a highly publicized affair sponsored by Canada's national airline. It was covered on nightly national television and was front page news back home for weeks. But when the deaths and dissension occurred, the press quickly dumped on the expedition, dubbing it a failure. Many Canadians wrote it off.

From the ashes of the expedition rose a phoenix. The remaining team members regrouped, rekindled their resolve and continued climbing. Within weeks, they had put not one but six team members on top of the world, the first of whom was Laurie. It was one of the most courageous comebacks ever recorded in Everest's long and dramatic history.

Laurie returned to Everest a second time in 1986 and was instrumental in assisting one of his climbing protégés, Canadian Sharon Wood, of Canmore, Alberta, in becoming the first North American woman to reach the summit.

Laurie's mental toughness and fortitude were well known. In the process of evacuating one of the bodies during the '82 expedition, Laurie had fallen into a crevasse and cracked three ribs. Although every breath was painful, he still managed to climb the mountain. At his core, he was a warrior. He had a fascination with guns, and if you were a friend, he regarded you as an ally in his army. An ally to Laurie meant he would come after you in a howling blizzard and find you no matter how long it took. He had always supported me in my own dream to climb Everest and he had done the same for all the other Canadians who had followed in his footsteps. He was a decent man and loyalty meant a lot to him.

But there was far more to Laurie than a mountaineer. He was a deeply philosophical person with an eccentric character. He believed in past lives, the wisdom of aboriginal Shamans and native spiritual customs.

Without saying a word, he sat down on my bed and gave me a long hug. I could hear his breathing in my ear and feel his energy coursing through me. I felt his thick leathered fingers envelop mine. He squeezed them with such force it hurt.

"You were once one of my legionnaires," he attested as his stare burned into me and he retreated to a place of spirituality deep inside himself. "We have fought battles together in past lives and now you are in a battle in this life. This is a fight for your life. This is a battle you must win. To win, you must focus all your energies on one thing and only one thing.

"There are only two ways off this ward. The first is they wheel your body down to the morgue on a stretcher. The second is you walk out of here under your own steam. So from this moment forward, decide which outcome you want. When you have, eliminate anything extraneous. Focus everything you have on this challenge."

Although I disagreed with Laurie's fight or die approach, I could not help but feel the passion and sincerity in his words. With a combination of awe and ambition, I listened as he drove his points home. His lips drew back across his face into a thin line, his eyes narrowed and his speech slowed. He spoke of character, of courage, of victory and defeat. And he spoke of hope – how and where to find it and how to nurture it in ourselves. When he finished, he wrapped me once again in his arms and whispered something in my ear I will never forget. "When we run away from fear, it gets bigger," he stated with conviction, "but when we advance towards it, it shrinks."

> *"When we run away from fear, it gets bigger,*
> *but when we advance towards it, it shrinks."*
>
> – Mr. Laurie Skreslet,
> First Canadian to Climb Mt. Everest

At that moment, I knew what I had to do. Reaching over to my side table, I opened a drawer and pulled out Valerie Simonson's pin. Then I carefully attached it to Laurie's vest.

"Focus all your energies and power through this pin," I said. "Thank you for brightening my day, Laurie. You are a fine man and a good friend. Bless you for coming."

After shaking hands with Eric and hugging Cecilia, Laurie did an about-face, slapped my clothes closet door with an emphatic whack of his hand and marched from the room as swiftly as he had come.

No one spoke for about a minute. The aura of Everest and the man who most personified what the mountain meant to me continued to electrify the room.

I looked out the window. On the other side of the pane I could see the lights of downtown Calgary shining in the distance. I told Cecilia and Eric how much I loved them and vowed to remember always what Laurie had told me.

Beyond the darkness, beyond the fear, the objective was now clear.

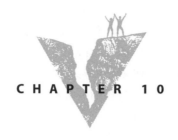

CHAPTER 10

Cecilia
DESPERATE MEASURES

Kitchens have always been places of joy in my life. When I was growing up in New Orleans, friends and family would gather in the kitchen to concoct delectable meals in the welcoming warmth of comfortable conversation. Seasonings and flavors came together in a gumbo of laughs. So much love went into those meals, and the food seemed to be all the more delicious because of the good spirits and kind intentions with which it was made. I remember those meals with a happy feeling in my heart.

The Unit 57 kitchen is as small as a closet. It reminds me of the tiny one in my efficiency apartment during my university days. There are no windows and only one entrance. As I walk in, the "General" refrigerator is on the right. Next to it is a small countertop with a toaster and cabinets above. To my left are a blender and microwave, as well as cabinets containing paper cups, napkins, coffee and tea. The "For Immune Suppressed Patients Only" refrigerator is in the corner. "WASH YOUR HANDS" signs are posted everywhere.

I open the General refrigerator. There are neatly stacked rows of plastic containers filled with red, yellow and orange JELL-O. There are juice cups too: apple, orange and cranberry. The freezer is filled with small, single-serving containers of ice cream, those cups with the little wooden spoons you used to get as a kid.

The refrigerator For Immune Suppressed Patients Only is emblazoned with a huge "WASH YOUR HANDS" sign. I recall our brief orientation on the process that might "cure" Alan of his leukemia. After each dose of chemotherapy, the patient's immune system becomes weaker and weaker. The treatment for Alan's form of leukemia is an adult blood stem cell transplant. This means they will strip his body of its entire immune system with high doses of chemotherapy. Just before transplant, Alan will have no immune system at all. This refrigerator is reserved for these patients.

We have decided that Alan is not to eat any of the hospital food. As is the case for most chemo patients, the very scent of the institutional food trays wafting down the hall makes him nauseous. Ever since those warm family meals back in Louisiana, I have believed that there is something special about having someone you love prepare food for you. In our case, it is crucial. Alan's food cannot originate in the hospital's bowels in a sterile, impersonal kitchen that leaches out all vitamins and minerals. To entice Alan to eat, I fix nutritious meals for him at home and take them to the hospital. I hope I also bring him the energy and appeal of food prepared with care and love.

Most mornings I come to the hospital with my backpack and cooler filled with what I hope will be his breakfast and lunch – watermelon wedges; baked potatoes I can cut, fry and serve with ketchup; and frozen blueberries and yogurt for making smoothies. Some days, he doesn't eat a thing, but settles for a few baked potato slices and if he's feeling ambitious, orange juice. His diet has always been excellent, so he's never really used supplements like vitamin pills and such even though at the moment it would probably be a good idea to take some. He eats very little red meat, mostly chicken and fish, and drinks no coffee, tea or alcohol. Eric jokes that we shouldn't put any stimulants into Alan because he's stimulated enough already. Alan rarely eats desserts and

I've never seen him drink a soft drink or eat any other kind of junk food, but he loves milk shakes, milk chocolate and hot chocolate. His favorite meal is baked chicken, mashed potatoes and corn on the cob, so that's one of the ones I prepare for him. Although he's rarely able to eat it all, he can usually force down the mashed potatoes. I try to mix in butter and parmesan cheese to increase the fat and protein content – anything to get more calories into him and minimize his weight loss. We're determined to keep his weight stable. He's got to eat. I see it as part of my responsibility to ensure he does.

My morning ritual involves following the life-preserving rules of the ward kitchen: washing my hands, unloading the containers from home carefully labeled with Alan's name, room number and the date, and placing them in the proper refrigerator.

I have carefully read all the manuals, pamphlets and internet information about the immune system and have determined that the best line of defense is a strong offense. I pledge that Alan will not get an infection if I have anything to do with it, especially not from the food I serve him. I sanitize his dishes and silverware at our apartment by immersing them in boiling water. I cook everything at the highest temperature and immediately wrap the food in aluminum foil. I set the package inside a heated pan and quickly drive to the hospital. There, I set out the placemat, silverware and glass at his bedside. With a hopeful smile, I lay out the food and turn to Alan.

I meet patients and caregivers in Unit 57's kitchen at all hours of the day and night. Cancer patients do not have a set time for meals. They eat what they can, when they can. The Unit 57 kitchen can manage only two or three people at a time. Often, I wait patiently for my turn to enter, always allowing patients to go ahead of me when they've worked up enough courage to eat.

Without exception, all the people who enter the kitchen have the same look of desperation in their eyes. A patient shuffles in with his I.V. lifeline and opens the refrigerator door. The cool air hits him in the face as he leans over and stares at the neatly stacked rows of colored containers, trying to will himself to take one. His childhood memories of the sweetness of JELL-O and ice cream are replaced with a metallic taste. If only he could enjoy the taste of these sweet snacks.

The caregivers too take their time peering into the refrigerator, looking for a loved one's containers. I find myself gazing into the light, looking for the container labeled HOBSON. *Where is that snack he didn't want this morning?*

When Alan expresses a desire for a milk shake, I jump at the chance to mix up something he will enjoy. I bounce down the hall with his favorite glass in hand, greeting several of the nurses along the way, declaring with a big smile on my face, "He wants a milk shake!" As I turn the corner to enter the kitchen, I suddenly see a woman with a knife in her hand stabbing a box of frozen strawberries. She must feel me staring at her because she swiftly turns to face me. With bloodshot eyes she says, "My daughter wants a strawberry smoothie."

For a moment, we are both silent. Our eyes express what words cannot – simple desperation. We are desperate to give our loved ones just one thing, anything they can eat and enjoy. We know they may only take one sip or bite, but to us that is enough.

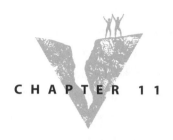

CHAPTER 11

Alan
CAMP
2

During my fifth night, things started to get a little more uncomfortable. After tossing around half-asleep for hours, I awoke to realize that my bed sheets were completely soaked. I rang for the night nurse to help me change them. When she arrived, I began to apologize for wetting the bed, but she swiftly cut me off.

"You didn't wet the bed, Alan," she reassured firmly. "You're having night sweats. Your body is sweating to try to counteract the heat created by the destruction of billions of cells inside you. You need to be gentler on yourself. This is a difficult process for anyone to go through. Just keep drinking water."

While I appreciated her wisdom and professionalism, another piece of my pride fell away at that moment. I remembered how my mother had changed my sheets when I had had a fever as a boy. Then I had felt relieved that someone I trusted had been there to take care of me. Now I felt like I had lost control of my body. I was a 42-year-old who needed to have his bed sheets changed. It was humbling.

As the days wore on, I began to approach Camp 3. On Everest, this is at about 24,000 feet, when you start to bump the top of your head against the bottom of "The Death Zone" where the pressure of the oxygen in the air is so low that it can only sustain life for very short periods of time. In Camp 3, it is very difficult to sleep, not only because of the altitude, but because of the sheer 2,000-foot drop just inches outside your tent. You need only zip open the front door to be reminded how close you are to death.

Peering over this precipice was like peering into the rooms of some of the other survivors on the ward. The tone in their enclaves was markedly subdued, and it signaled the severity of the struggle for life as graphically as the empty expanse of air beneath Camp 3. Inside those tents on 57, the climb had been going on for weeks, months and sometimes years, and the climbers and support team members were approaching exhaustion. Looking through the doors, you could feel the energy being sucked into the void the way breath vaporized into the cold, thin air at high altitude.

Thankfully, because it was early in our climb, our team was still fresh. That morning, Cecilia arrived smiling and radiant, toting a backpack of supplies and a cooler full of food. "Good morning, sweetie," she said, giving me a tender kiss and a warm hug. "How was your night?" She greeted me like this every morning. The nurses immediately took note of it and praised her for her strength and commitment. In her typical Louisiana fashion, she just smiled warmly and paid them a compliment in return. The rippling waves of her positive energy rolled out to others and then back to herself. She spread light wherever she went even if things were sometimes dark.

When Cecilia inquired what I wished for breakfast, I would usually emerge from my lethargy to say, "Nothing thanks, my love." She would ignore this and usually convince me to start with something bland like a baked potato.

"Super C" and "Cecilia Sherpa" as I came to call her, flatly refused to let me miss a meal or the nibble we called a meal. Every morning, she would check my weight on the wall calendar Bolek had created. If it had dropped, we would redouble our commitment to eat everything I could force down and hold down. This required constant diligence. The only way to hope to create a future was to act with as much fervor as possible in the present.

I went everywhere with my little black waist pack. Every time I passed another survivor in the hall or walked by a survivor's room, I was reminded of how fortunate I was to have my physical freedom. Many of them were much further along in the treatment process or had been admitted in far worse condition than I, and as a result, were markedly weaker. I tried not to think about how long it would be until I joined them. This was a constant difficulty. It was so easy to let my mind race away into the past to mourn what I had lost, or into the future to imagine all manner of horrible outcomes. But whether I looked forward or back, my conclusion was the same – I could no more change the past now than I could have before my illness. And I had equally little control over the future. The only thing I could control was my present – my present thoughts, feelings and actions. So, I retreated increasingly within myself, seeking solitude in silence and meditation. It was the only place where my mental chatter seemed to stop or at least slow down. I lived in the moment.

By now I was starting to get used to the daily routine on 57: housekeeping at 7 a.m., patient weighing at 8, breakfast at 9 and rounds at 10. Outside each room, the resident, attending physician, charge nurse and sometimes a few medical students would huddle to discuss the condition of the patient they were about to visit. Whenever I heard that "the pack" was starting its way down my wing of the ward, I would make sure to stay close to my room until the powwow arrived. The result of rounds often determined if I could go home on a day or overnight pass. From my point of view, even after a few days in hospital, any kind of pass was like a furlough from prison.

After rounds, I tried to haul myself to the ward's stationary bike for a little physical activity. It was there that I first met a man who would figure prominently in my future.

Dr. Jim Russell stood a little over five feet. He appeared before me in a white lab coat, pockets stuffed with notepads, pens and a stethoscope, and he lounged against the windows in front of the bike sunning himself like a cat. He held his reading glasses by one end and spun them around like a cowboy spinning a lasso. Peering at me curiously beneath a thick shock of short dark hair, he extended his hand and declared in a crisp English accent: "Hello, Alan. The name's Jim. I understand you climb mountains."

"I have in the past," I acknowledged, "but whether I will again remains a mystery at the moment."

"I can understand that," he agreed. "We're going to see if we can do something about that. What's life without a bit of mystery, anyway?"

Jim's manner was disarming and the twinkle in his eye captivating. He went on to calmly explain a little about the adult blood stem cell transplant process, then bid me a pleasant goodbye and left me to my labors on the bike.

"Cheerio," he said as he headed off to see another survivor.

A native of Sussex, England, Jim Russell was the oncologist who headed up the adult blood stem cell and bone marrow transplant team at the Foothills Medical Centre. He was also one of the world's finest blood and bone marrow transplanters. For twelve years, he had been Director of the Alberta Bone Marrow and Blood Cell Transplant Program. His easy-going, down-to-earth nature veiled his deep competence, vast experience and massive knowledge. In recent years, he had earned the nickname "The Cowboy" as a man who thought outside the box. He had been amongst the first in the world, for example, to abolish the practice of isolating adult blood cell and bone marrow transplant recipients in plastic tents to protect them from possible infection. He deemed this practice unnecessary. Alberta's dry climate made the likelihood of potentially lethal fungal infections highly improbable. He also believed the practice was psychologically devastating to patients and was more detrimental to their mental and emotional health than the potential risk of any infection. This holistic view of patients had established Jim as a man of deep compassion who treated not only an illness, but the entire individual.

That day, my introduction to Jim was brief, but significant. I would eventually become one of his patients and come to know him well. During our first meeting and the many that followed, his behavior and demeanor were absolutely consistent. He never introduced himself as "Dr. Russell," only Jim. Unpretentious and quiet, he had an arid sense of humor and a childlike playfulness. Perceptive and sensitive to the needs of others, Jim was a natural leader. Yet he always led from behind and pushed others to the front. He may have been an elite doctor, but he was not an elitist. He was a loveable "chap." Cecilia and I called him "Gentle Jim."

Later that afternoon, I received my first Reiki treatment. Reiki, the laying-on of hands, is a form of Japanese energy channeling and relaxation (*Rei* means "universal"; *ki* is "life force energy"). Although it is a millennia-old healing system with probable roots in ancient Tibet, it was introduced to the West only in the 1930s in Hawaii. In theory, it works by helping remove toxic energy and substances, whether physical, mental, emotional or spiritual. During treatments, practitioners use their hands to redirect healing energy from a Higher Power through their own bodies and radiate it into the patient. In return, they may also pick up negative energy from the patient and send it off into the air. Without a vessel such as a body to contain it, the energy quickly dissipates. There are now an estimated fifty thousand Reiki Masters worldwide and as many as a million people practicing the art.

My healers that day were Patti Mayer; Jane Stewart, the managing director of The Alternative Cancer Research Foundation; and Mary Tidlund, a successful businesswoman turned philanthropist. To the sound of soothing music from my tape player, each of them took turns holding their hands just inches from my head, feet, shoulders and stomach. As I drifted off into deep meditation with my eyes closed, they periodically rotated their positions until they had successfully "removed" as much excess heat from my body as possible.

Reiki sessions appear deceptively simple to an outside observer. Skeptics scoff at Reiki, claiming it is quackery. But from my point of view as a survivor, I found it to be greatly restorative. Not only did I get a chance to disappear from the world, fall into a semi-sleep and escape from the reality of life-threatening illness for a few minutes, but when the sessions were over, I felt relaxed and energized. The presence of Patti, Jane and Mary, each of whom exuded calm and peace, served to magnify the purity of the experience. Here were three very busy professionals who had given freely of their time and expertise to attend to the needs of another. Even if the procedure had had no effect, I would have considered their presence alone valuable enough. But during the sessions, it was as if a very hot and heavy weight was somehow lifted from my body. If this was quackery, I wanted more of it. Each treatment lasted about forty-five minutes, but it had such significant effects that it felt like three hours. During the sessions, the nursing staff respected my personal space and we were not disturbed. I emerged substantially refreshed.

"Wow!" I enthused after the treatment. "That was incredible. I don't know what you guys did, but I feel a whole lot lighter."

"We felt fire coming out of your body," Jane revealed. "I could feel my hands getting hotter and hotter, but when I shook them off into the air, I could take more. It was an amazing experience."

"What do I owe you?" I asked as the trio was leaving.

"Nothing but a smile," Mary replied, "and every effort you can make to get back to full health."

"I can do that," I promised, "and then some. Thanks for coming and cooling things down around here. It was getting a little heated."

They all laughed, each gave me a hug and a kiss and promised to return whenever I wished.

Later that afternoon, I changed rooms yet again, this time to across the hall and a few doors down. This regular inconvenience was the consequence of the ever-shifting landscape of life on the ward – new patients being admitted, others being discharged. Still others required private rooms when their immune systems became so depleted by chemo that they could no longer risk exposure to the germs and viruses carried by others. I soon got used to this little game of musical rooms and learned to accept it. All of the rooms were basically the same, but the constant shifting of my perspective actually helped prevent me from feeling like I would be there for the rest of my life.

Unit 57 bustled. There were always visitors coming and going, survivors being accompanied to diagnostic tests and procedures on and off the ward, announcements being made, and nurses, doctors, porters, personal care assistants, psychologists, pharmacists, dieticians, physiotherapists, housekeepers, students and researchers scurrying around at all times of the day and night. My previous vision of a ward as a staid, sanitized and strictly regimented place in which sick people just lay around idly in beds evaporated in those first few days on the unit. What replaced this view was wonder at the complexity and constant change. A whole lot of people were hustling to do a whole lot of work in a very big hurry. While the patients may have had the sense things were moving slowly, you had only to walk by the nursing station anytime during the day shift to witness the lively dynamic of acute care in action. Implicitly, everyone understood that death's door was just at the end of the corridor. The objective was to keep that door from opening before its time.

Early that evening, Eric made another visit, this time accompanied by our cousin, Bob McKenzie. Bob is a skyscraper of a man, standing over 6 feet 4 inches. Although middle-aged, he still has a youthful face and a great sense of adventure. I had always been impressed by Bob, not so much by his considerable business skills, but by his interpersonal ones. He listened intently and empathized instantly.

"So, what do you need in here?" he asked after a while, looking around the room. "This place could get to feel confining pretty quickly."

"To tell you the truth, Bob," I admitted, "I haven't had time to let it grow on me and I don't plan on being in here long enough to let it get that way either."

"Let's just make sure it stays that way…We'll be back tomorrow," he promised. His eyes danced mysteriously as they left.

The next day Bob was back, this time with a computer programmed by his son, Brian, so I could log onto the internet. He also carted in a brand new bar refrigerator and proceeded to pack it full of boxes of fruit juice.

"There," he observed after about half an hour of effort. "That should keep your body fed and your intellect stimulated so you don't unplug from the world in here. As for food for your soul, we'll leave that to Cecilia."

I started to cry. I wondered where all the humanity came from. I gave Bob a big hug.

"Why?" I asked him. "Why me?"

"My grandmother once told me that good folk are few," he reflected after a while. "When you find them, keep them, nurture them. They are precious."

Then he left.

I thought about what had just happened. I was again struck by the juxtapositions cancer created – on one hand paralyzing fear, on the other incredible compassion. It brought out the best and worst in those whose lives it touched.

By now, I was pining to get outside. I had been in hospital for six days, and Cecilia and I had been planning a quick escape. We had successfully negotiated for a pass so we could go out for dinner that evening. So far, my white blood cell counts were not low enough to prevent me from leaving the hospital and eating normal food, so Super C and I packed up our car and hit the road with great expectancy.

While we were driving west at sunset, I rolled down the window of the passenger side and like a dog, experienced the glory of the air jetting through my nostrils. It was fantastic to finally breathe outside air. It was equally magnificent to feel the wind in my hair. I was not sure how much longer I would have that luxury, so I relished it. In the distance, I could see the silhouette of the Canadian Rockies against the blazing fireball of the setting sun. Beyond that I knew was our ultimate goal – the freedom of the hills.

On the edge of the city, we pulled into the parking lot of a small restaurant. I leaped out of the front seat anticipating the sweet taste of freedom only moments away, but suddenly, it was foreshortened.

I got just six inches out of the seat when my I.V. line caught on a lever beneath it. My central line was yanked violently downwards and I felt an intense burning sensation in my chest. In an instant, I folded back into the car, doubled over in pain.

Cecilia could do nothing but watch and pray the blood would not start gushing from my chest. For a minute, I writhed in agony waiting for the spurting to start.

We never made it to the restaurant that day. We drove straight back to the hospital and headed directly to my room. Fortunately, my line stayed in place and the bleeding never started. But days later, I would pay dearly for our moment of exuberance.

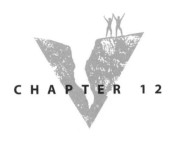

C H A P T E R   1 2

Cecilia

H E A L E R S

The range of healers supporting us is remarkable. We are using everything western medicine has to offer, and so much more. This has been true since our first moments at the hospital when Patti Mayer cleared the room of negative energy. It was my first glimpse of healing beyond convention.

Today, I am carefully writing down the telephone messages Alan receives from friends on his voicemail. One lovely voice says, "Hi, I'm Mary. Patti Mayer thought Alan might benefit from a Reiki session. When can we come by?" I have to play the message back several times before I can understand what she's saying. What kind of a session? How do you spell that? Luckily, I am at the office and can immediately jump on the internet. I find out that Reiki is a channeling of energy. It sounds interesting, so I read more. Apparently, it has a positive effect on many forms of illness and other negative conditions. The side effects of medical treatments such as chemotherapy can be reduced or eliminated with Reiki treatments, the information says.

If there is something to help Alan deal with chemo treatments, I'm all for it. It was terrible watching my Mom suffer through hers. I can't wait to give Alan the message and schedule his first Reiki session.

On the appointed day, Mary Tidlund, Jane Stewart and Patti arrive promptly at 11 a.m. The nurses have been told of the treatment and they have posted a "Do Not Disturb" sign on Alan's door. I think this is very accommodating. Part of me wants to stay and watch, but another wants to just let whatever needs to happen, happen.

I leave Alan lying on the bed with Mary and Jane standing on either side of him and Patti at his head. They have not yet started, but I can feel an energy in the room I haven't felt before. I sense he is in good hands and feel at ease leaving him in their care. Something good is about to happen.

I head down to the cafeteria for a cup of tea and try to imagine what might be happening in the room. After an hour, I return. Mary, Jane and Patti are gone. I give Alan a kiss on the forehead and ask, "How was it? How do you feel? What did they do?" Alan replies in a calm, steady voice, "I feel wonderful – relaxed, at peace and believe it or not, carefree." Incredible, I think, for Alan to say something like that and be so serene. Something must have happened. I would like to have this feeling too. Perhaps I can have some Reiki treatments too.

Mary, Jane and Patti return several times during Alan's hospital stay. Later, Patti also arranges for Alan to see Dr. Steven Aung, a Chinese Master Healer. He prescribes various Chinese herbs to boost Alan's immune system and improve his energy and kidney function. Chemotherapy drugs are expelled from the body in urine produced by the kidneys. The chemo is hard on them.

At first, I am a bit concerned. I wonder whether the herbs might work against the chemo treatments he is receiving or cause an adverse reaction. I expect the doctors and nurses to discourage the use of such supplements, but to my surprise, they welcome this complementary form of treatment. With their approval, I feel relieved.

Alan's meditation instructor, Valerie Simonson, is another healer who blesses us. When I return home at night and nestle into bed, I reach for my sleeping aid, a meditation tape I had purchased from the local

Brahma Kumaris Meditation Centre. Valerie introduced us to open eye meditation when I first came to Calgary. There are many nights when I play meditation tapes for hours while I try to relax. I find one tape particularly useful in helping me fall asleep. After a full day at the hospital, my mind reels with "what ifs." My body is filled with anxiety.

I turn off the lights and put the tape into the tape player on the nightstand. While peaceful music plays in the background, a soft soothing female voice says...

Let me imagine that nothing exists outside this room

I feel completely insulated from the outside world

I turn all my attention inward,
concentrating my thought energy on the center of the forehead

I feel a sense of detachment from my physical body
and the physical surroundings

I become aware of the stillness around me and within me

A feeling of natural peacefulness begins to steal over me

Waves of peace gently wash over me, removing any restlessness
and tension from my mind

I concentrate on this feeling of deep peace

Just peace

I am peace

Peace is my true state of being

My mind becomes very calm and clear

I feel easy and content

Having returned to my natural consciousness of peace

I lie for a while, enjoying this feeling of calmness and serenity...

– Practical Meditation,
Brahma Kumaris World Spiritual University,
London

3rd Tool for *Caregivers*
Manage Your Mind

Some nights, I drift off to sleep before the tape ends. On other nights, it is more difficult and I have to replay the tape several times before I am finally able to nod off. During those nights when I listen to the tape, my dreams are comforting and I awake feeling rested.

CHAPTER 13

Alan
CAMP
3

"Our perception of reality is frequently much worse than reality itself. I'm always better – always – at imagining the doom and gloom and the unsuccessful steps before I imagine the successful outcome. So I have to counter that, and the way I counter it is through rational thought, instead of just an emotional reaction. If I were just to react all the time, I would never take risks. But to take action is a counter-reaction."

– Sharon Wood,
First North American Woman to Climb Mt. Everest,
One Step Beyond

I laid quietly in the sunshine across the road from the hospital letting the fresh air wash over my face like a breaking wave of cool, clear water. I ran my fingers slowly through the green grass under the tree, treasuring the sensation. Ah, to be outside, to be free, to be alive. I listened to the wind rustle the leaves above. I drew the air through my nostrils in long deep breaths.

It happens so infrequently in life that we have moments like this, moments of peace when the bustle of the day melts away and we realize we have been looking in the wrong place. Happiness is not far away. It is every day. The feeling can wind its way gently into our psyche and then quietly perch itself like a bird alighting on a branch. There, it can cock its head toward us and in a sweet song hail us to stop long enough to get back in touch with ourselves. It is there, not at the movies or the theme parks or the "happy hours," that true joy and happiness actually exist. It is not an act of doing. It is an act of being.

Cecilia and I cuddled in the sun. Chemo disappeared, leukemia took flight, and a Higher Power took hold. Neither one of us wanted to return to the ward. We just wanted to stay there holding each other forever, delighting in the moment. Later, we would return to that moment again and again, recreating it in our minds. The days were filled with so many unsettling moments and thoughts that we needed a safe place to return to – even if that place was in our heads.

At the appointed hour for my next medication, we returned somberly to the ward. There was a discipline involved in following the treatment protocol and we had to stick with the program. Getting better was a full-time job.

The final two days of "juice" came and went without incident. I continued to receive many visitors. I fed off their energy, storing it like a squirrel does nuts for the upcoming winter. Cecilia and I knew that as the newness of our situation wore off, we would be faced with the reality of many long hours and days alone with only our thoughts. For the moment, however, our days were filled with love and companionship.

The day after my first wave of chemo ended, we got our first full-day pass to go home. It was glorious. As soon as rounds and meds were over, Cecilia and I were out of there in no time. We drove home to our apartment and I immediately went to bed. Within minutes, I fell into a blissful sleep. For three hours, the world vanished. After a light dinner, we returned to the hospital at 8 p.m. for an infusion of antibiotics. So began the next phase in my treatment.

As the chemo continued to do its work over the coming days and weeks, the strength of my immune system declined daily. Without what I called "my immune system in a bag" – the I.V. antibiotics – I would not survive. At the same time, my red blood cells, white blood cells and platelets were being destroyed. I would receive regular transfusions when my levels became too low. These precious blood products came from completely anonymous donors to whose generosity I owe my life.

Cecilia and I were now walking a deadly tightrope. With every passing day, my blood cell counts plummeted further. For the first few days after chemo, I was allowed to come and go from the hospital during the day as long as I came back for antibiotics and units of red blood cells and platelets each evening. The nurses and Cecilia watched me closely.

"If his temperature hits 100 degrees [F]," the nurses advised, "get back in here immediately. It's much easier to catch an infection than to chase it."

A couple of days later, my mother arrived from eastern Canada. Isabel Hobson was about my height, five foot six, with brown hair that reached between her shoulder blades. She had graduated at the top of her university class and had an incredible memory for names, faces and relationships. Her official degree was in physical education, but she had an informal Ph.D. in parenting. While I was growing up, my father had put in twelve-hour days as a research scientist, and she had toiled tirelessly at home, preparing meals, doing laundry, shopping for groceries and ferrying me and my three brothers to and from our activities – everything from skiing and swimming to gymnastics, tennis and badminton. As a teenager, I had once watched in astonishment as she single-handedly dragged a fully laden, two hundred pound canoe up and over a four foot high beaver dam after my father and I suddenly slipped at the moment we were supposed to be pushing. Together with my Dad, she had successfully put all four boys through university. Later in life, as a middle-aged empty-nester, she had boldly returned to work as an executive assistant with the federal government. At the same time, she had become extensively involved in Project Ploughshares, an international organization dedicated to world peace and environmental issues. In short, she was a strong-willed, emotionally sensitive and impressive woman with a passion for her family, her friends and the planet.

It was wonderful to see Mum, but unfortunately, there was little she could do but watch. Heaven knows what she must have been thinking. First, one of her grandsons dies of leukemia, a second narrowly escapes it and now her own son faces the same menace. It must have been hard for her to see me as the latest one in a hospital bed.

By now, I had little energy left for anyone save myself. Mum wanted desperately to help, but she had to settle for just sitting and chatting. After a while, I had limited energy even for that.

That afternoon, we got a call from my nephew, Michael, in Vancouver. He had been through a bone marrow transplant six years earlier. I remembered speaking to him via satellite from high on Everest. His struggles in the hospital at the time had made ours on the mountain seem inconsequential. We, after all, had volunteered and trained for our climb. He had had no time to prepare for his. Who would have thought that six years later our roles would be reversed? Michael reminded me that my day of diagnosis had been his late brother's birthday. That gave me the shivers.

"Now you hang in there, Uncle Alan," he urged. "We believe in you and love you very much."

"I love you, too," I declared. "You are one tough guy, Michael, and I am only now beginning to realize exactly how tough."

> *Every few weeks, I'd call Michael to see how he was doing on his mountain…I remember hanging up from those calls and thinking that despite our challenges, we were lucky to be alive. We hadn't been relegated to a hospital bed by some cruel genetic twist. We were living our dreams.*
>
> *– The Triumph of Tenacity*
> *(formerly titled, The Power of Passion)*

Two days later, as I lay quietly in my hospital bed, I was struck with a commanding thought. It started slowly, then gradually grew stronger until suddenly and inexplicably, it spilled out of my mouth.

"It's Eric," I said.

"What did you say?" Cecilia asked.

"I said, 'It's Eric.'"

"What do you mean, 'It's Eric'?" she countered. "What's Eric?"

"The donor's Eric, Cecilia," I clarified. "It just hit me. The donor's Eric. I feel it. I know it."

"That would be fabulous if it was Eric," she agreed as she came over and sat next to me. "You so admire him, and it would be such a great chance to create a closer bond between the two of you. It really would be wonderful."

"It *is* wonderful," I reiterated. "That is the absolute marvel of it all. It's Eric. Can you write it down somewhere?"

"Absolutely, sweetie," she said.

She did. It was August 23 – thirty-nine months to the day that I had stood on the top of Everest at age thirty-nine.

Cecilia and I did not speak of my premonition again, but at that moment something inside me began to change. I felt like more weight was starting to be taken off my shoulders and that somehow, somewhere, there was something larger going on that involved me and yet had nothing to do with me. It was not wishful thinking. Nor was it the desperate prayer of a desperate man. It was simply a message I received, verbalized and then thanks to the shortcomings of the human mind, quickly set aside as implausible. It was too good to be true.

At about the same time, Eric had exactly the same premonition. As soon as the search for a donor began, his wife, Diane, had told him: "You're going to be the one." Eric had replied, "It's funny, but I get the same feeling."

The next day, I began to feel unwell and thought it best to stay close to the hospital. My central line was beginning to feel uncomfortable. The skin around the entry point had become red and sore. I thought this was probably just the result of having almost yanked it from its socket, but to be on the safe side, the doctors decided to take a blood culture to test for infection. If the central line had indeed become infected, it might have grave consequences for me. Any little bug living in it could be mainlined throughout my body within seconds, and with no immune system to combat it, I might quickly die.

By the end of the week, I had spiked a fever. Cecilia rushed me to the hospital. She kept a vigil at my bedside fourteen hours a day.

I learned early in my hospitalization that when it comes to leukemia, the medical profession takes even the hint of a potential infection very seriously. Rather than wait to determine if it is bacterial, viral or fungal, they hit you hard and fast with everything they have.

First, I received a visit from Rob Tingley, a member of the hospital's Infectious Diseases Unit. When he arrived on the ward, I was squatted on the floor in front of the elevator holding my head between my legs, struggling through a headache. Because we had never met before, he inadvertently swept by me and into my room, which was right next to the elevator. A moment later, he reappeared looking perplexed.

"Are you looking for Alan Hobson by any chance?" I inquired, deducing who he was.

His head spun around trying to figure out where the voice was coming from.

"If you're with infectious diseases," I continued, not lifting my head from its bowed position, "I'm probably your man."

Rob approached me slowly.

"Oh, you're Alan," he observed. "Sorry to see you're not feeling well. We need to talk."

"Great," I remarked. "Unfortunately, it's going to have to take place while we walk outside because it took me a lot of effort just to get to the elevator."

"Fine," Rob assented. "You lead."

Cecilia, Rob and I got into the elevator, rode it down to the main floor and then walked out into the sunshine. As soon as I breathed my first lungful of outside air, my headache abated significantly. We walked straight toward the back of the hospital.

"For a guy with a hemoglobin level down in the sidewalk, you're doing pretty well," Rob commented.

"I appreciate the compliment," I said, "but just don't ask me to stop. If I do, I might not get started again."

Rob, a young and enthusiastic clinician, knew a lot about infectious diseases. We talked about my central line and my greatest fear – that the horrendous bugs I had invariably picked up in the developing world during my expeditions might still be living in my guts after chemo. If the little devils were still breathing, I might not stand much of a chance if they multiplied.

"We don't know what's happening yet," Rob advised carefully, "but with your permission, I'm going to recommend we start you on an anti-fungal agent right away."

The deadliest of all infections and the one most dreaded in a leukemia patient is a fungal infection. This is why plants and flowers are not allowed on the ward. The soil in which they are grown can contain spores and fungi that could prove lethal to anyone with a seriously depleted immune system. To such a person, a fungal infection is the equivalent of a forest fire that can quickly get out of control. The only solution is to hit you the metaphorical water bombers.

The water bomber has a name. They call it amphotericin. The nurses called it "ampho-terrible" and it did not take me long to figure out why.

They brought it into my room in a brown paper bag a few hours after Rob had gone.

"What's that?" I asked. "A bottle of cheap wine?"

"No, Alan, it isn't," the nurse replied wryly. "This is amphotericin. The reason it's in a brown paper bag is to ensure its contents don't react with light."

"So it's like mushrooms," I remarked. "It grows best when it's kept in the dark."

"Something like that," the nurse replied, trying to ignore my cheekiness.

The tone in the room swiftly began to change. The nurse explained that she would start with a short preliminary test to see how my body reacted to the medication. If there were no side effects, she would increase the dosage.

The greatest potential side effect of amphotericin is kidney failure, but more common is something called "rigors." Not to be confused with rigor mortis, rigors are like an internal earthquake, an uncontrolled shaking that can become so violent that patients sometimes fall out of bed. Their respiration rate rockets, they feel intensely chilled and they are unable to calm their breathing or still their shuddering bodies. It can be terrifying.

I passed the first test with no ill effects. I visualized the medication as warm mushroom soup and that seemed to help. Perhaps it was the magic of the mind-body connection again, or maybe it was simply good luck. Whatever it was, it was a relief to have the test completed. Unfortunately, that also meant that the nurse was clear to give me a higher dose. As the ampho began to run through me, I was confined to my room.

For the past several days, I had awakened each morning to find more and more of my hair on my pillow. It was now starting to fall out in clumps. Cecilia suggested that now might be a good time to shave my head rather than wait for all my hair to fall out. She disappeared to find my nurse, Michael Bonnaventure.

The decision to shave your head is a pivotal rite of passage for any chemotherapy patient. It is far more than a physical act. It is a deeply personal commitment to expose yourself as you have not been exposed since birth. It calls into question significant issues concerning how we perceive ourselves and how others perceive us.

Like it or not, most of us in the developed world have accepted the stereotype that we must be, or we must appear to be, young, energetic, attractive, enthusiastic, intelligent, healthy, wealthy, physically fit, mentally, spiritually and emotionally balanced, successful, happy and fulfilled. This utopia, of course, is almost unattainable, especially with any permanence. The harder we seek it, the more it eludes us.

That is why the simple act of losing our hair can communicate beyond words that which we most dread – that we may be old, tired, unattractive and unwell. We may respond, as I did, by wearing bandannas and hats, or in the case of many women, wigs and turbans. These do more than help insulate us from the cold (and it is absolutely amazing how much insulation a little hair offers compared to a completely bald head). They help us protect our already shaken self-image from societal stigmas and enable us to maintain the appearance that we are still in control of our lives and our bodies. Cancer attacks our self-identity, and this, perhaps more than the side effects of chemotherapy, radiation or surgery, is one of the biggest dilemmas the disease presents.

Contemplating the answer to the question "Who am I?" can be terrifying, but answering it can be invaluable. If we can somehow see past life-threatening illness as something that steals away who we are and instead see it as something that strips away who we are not, we may come closer to some of the value in the experience. Just as Michelangelo believed that his sculpture of the statue of David had always been locked in the marble and he had only to remove the stone around it, so it is that cancer can reveal the essence of who we are separate from our bodies.

At the moment of trying to decide whether or not to have my head shaved, I was a long way from knowing this. I was too caught up in my physical appearance to understand that what I saw in the mirror was not actually who I was. I was not my body. My body was simply the house in which I was temporarily living. The hair on the top of the house, like the shingles on the roof, was matted lifelessly to it. I knew it was only a matter of time before the remaining strands fell out completely.

Solemnly, I gave Michael the nod. He went to find Denny Netik, a personal care assistant, the man with the shears. Minutes later, the pair returned and started work.

The process took only a few minutes. To their credit, Michael and Denny handled the whole thing lightly and easily. When it was over, I lay back on the bed, afraid to sit up and peer at my reflection. I did not want to see any ugly cranial imperfections I had never known about before. More than that, I did not want to see with my own eyes the external manifestation of what I already knew – that I had cancer. In that unsettling moment, I knew I would not only see, but I would actually *know*.

I did not want to know. I wanted this whole damn thing to go away. What was happening to me? Who were these men standing over me, what were they doing here and more importantly, what was *I* doing here? If I was not my body, who was *I*?

After five minutes of lying there fixated on the ceiling, I could not bear the suspense any longer. So I asked Cecilia for a hand mirror.

Holy shit! *Who is that? Is that me? Is that cancer? Or is that me with cancer?*

Not quite yes to all questions.

Quickly, I lay back down and looked up at the ceiling again.

"You look good with no hair," Cecilia complimented lovingly as she ran her fingers over my newly bald head. "You have a beautifully shaped head, sweetie."

Slowly, she bent over me and kissed my nakedness. I felt defenseless and bare.

By now the ampho had been running for a few hours. I went about my usual business of staying active on the ward, walking about and visiting here and there. Around 8 p.m., I began to feel very out-of-sorts. Cecilia and I returned to my room and I lay down.

I had been there only a few minutes when I began to feel chilled. Thinking it was just another wave of fever, I crawled under the covers, but within minutes my condition deteriorated from a shiver to a shake to a quake.

"Look out!" I cried out to Cecilia. "Here we go."

Cecilia pounced on me like a mother cat protecting a kitten. As my respiration started to increase, I could hear her breathing in my ear. Instantly, she rang for the nurse.

"Rigors in 86!" she yelled into the intercom.

Within seconds, Michael was in the room.

"Okay, Al," he reassured swiftly, but calmly. "This is just a reaction to the ampho. We're going to get you some Demerol immediately. Here come some hot blankets, buddy."

As my bed began to creak violently with my movements, Cecilia slid off my back. I could feel a wave of warm blankets envelop me. She moved briskly to tuck them tightly around me. This helped somewhat, but I felt like my body was being exorcised. It was completely rigid, vibrating recklessly. My respiration was racing.

"Okay Al," Mike shouted loudly so I could hear him over my breathing. "We've got your Demerol here and it's going up on the pole…I'm opening the valve now so it can flow into you…You'll begin to feel the calming effect in a few seconds…Hang in there, buddy. We've got you. It's going to be okay, Al. It's going to be okay."

Michael and Cecilia held me as my world imploded. I focused only on my breathing, trying in vain to calm myself, thinking of my meditation point and saying to myself, "C'mon, Baba. Give me your best stuff here, Pal. Stay with me. I'm not ready yet. I'm not going."

"Okay, Al," Michael soothed. "You should start to feel your body relaxing now. It's coming, Al…It's coming…"

Within a minute, my rigid muscles relaxed just a bit. The speed of my breathing began to abate. I continued to shake for a few minutes, then I settled into a shiver and finally into stillness. The storm was over.

This was our first real experience with what might be called trauma. Cecilia and I marveled at the strength and composure of the staff. The room became quiet. Gradually, I reconnected with my limbs.

"That was quite a ride," I confessed to Cecilia. "It was like going to another planet. I never want to go there again."

"You won't have to," Michael interjected. "We'll pre-medicate you next time with Benadryl. That should prevent the reaction."

"I hope so," I prayed as I clutched Cecilia. I thanked Baba for answering my call.

That night was rough. I felt like I had been stuffed into a paint mixer, shaken vigorously and my insides had burst. Psychologically, parts of me were still splattered on the ceiling, others on the window. It took time for me to collect myself. I was a mess.

The next day, my fever continued. I lay around partially dazed for most of the day. One moment I looked up to see one of the housekeepers, Derek Holt, standing over me with a mop on his head.

"Vood u like a 'ead buff?" he ventured in a mock French accent. "I vood be 'appy to oblige."

We laughed. It was great to let go. It had been quite a struggle.

The next morning was a pivotal one in my life. We received a message from Dr. Poon's office that we were to call. Apprehensively, Cecilia made her way to a phone at the end of the corridor. I stayed in bed, fearing the worst – more cancer.

A few minutes later, she burst back into the room.

"Eric's a match!" she exclaimed joyously. "Eric's a match!"

"You're kidding me?" I quavered. "You're kidding me!"

"I'm not," she retorted. "Eric's a full match – eight on eight parameters!"

"Holy shoot!" I marveled. "So it was true. I wasn't imagining things."

"No you weren't, sweetie," she cried, engulfing me in her arms. "It's true!"

The dam burst. Tears began to stream down my face as little sobs of elation sprang forth. A wave of euphoria poured over me the likes of which I had never experienced before. I let the emotions flow, closing my eyes and letting myself fall into them. I was weightless and peaceful and free, floating on a surge of possibility.

Cecilia held me as I cried. Together, we celebrated life and miracles and wonder.

Aside from love, hope was the most powerful medicine of all.

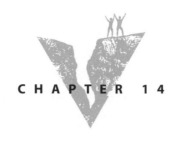

C H A P T E R   1 4

Cecilia
L O W S   A N D
H I G H S

If clothes define a man, then Alan is not a hospital patient. While the doctors wear their white lab coats and the nurses their brightly colored uniforms, Alan wears his casual clothes. He will not hear of wearing a hospital gown or slippers. His daily attire includes shorts and a T-shirt in summer and sweatpants and his favorite sweatshirt in winter.

Alan prepares for his fitness training at the hospital just as he does for training at home. He fills his plastic water bladder backpack (called a Camelbak), straps on his Polar heart rate monitor and pulls his sweatband over his brow. Wearing his white tank top, blue running shorts, white sports socks and running shoes, he departs for the "gym."

Off to one end of the ward, there is a sitting area with a lone stationary bike and treadmill. The equipment faces east toward the high-rise buildings of downtown. There is no humming of equipment beneath the beat of music, no televisions hanging from the ceilings, no other sweaty bodies synchronized in movement in a row of treadmills, but the picture of Alan on the stationary bike is the same to me. His face begins to flush from the exertion. His calves bulge with each pedal stroke. I marvel at his strength and discipline to exercise while his body is struggling with the chemo rushing through his body.

Alan is receiving continuous twenty-four hour chemotherapy, but you would never know it from looking at him. The nurses went out of their way to find a waist pack large enough to hold Alan's bag of chemo. While other survivors are walking around with their I.V. poles by their sides, Alan is self-contained. I see him as others see him – as an athlete in training.

We are now two weeks into his treatment and the side effects of chemo are starting to show. With a weak immune system, Alan is prone to fevers and infections. His hair has started to fall out. When I take his T-shirts home to wash, I notice blond strands clinging to them. I wonder what Alan will look like without hair. Will his head be round and evenly shaped or bumpy and rough? I have seen him in the tight black cap he wears in cold weather. I've also seen him in his white swimming cap. Both reveal a smoothly shaped head. I imagine his bald head will look no different.

I remember the shock of seeing my mother without hair. It seemed to happen all at once. One day, she had a full head of shiny black hair cut neatly to complement the round cheeks of her face. The next day, there were only scattered clumps, protruding out like the hair of a worn doll I played with as a child. My mother quickly went out and purchased a wig. I never liked it. I guess it wasn't actually the wig I disliked but what it represented to me. It concealed her baldness, but it could not hide her illness. She never spoke to me about her disease. Perhaps she wanted to protect me from reality, but her behavior only kept me distant and afraid.

Alan has been running a fever for twenty-four hours and the medical team is concerned that it might be a fungal infection. Fear sets in as a clinician with the hospital's Infectious Diseases Unit recommends starting Alan on an anti-fungal drug, amphotericin. The most common side effect of the medication is something called "rigors."

"Rigors? What's that?" I ask.

The clinician explains it's what happens when the patient's body senses that it's cold and starts rapidly contracting and relaxing its muscles to generate heat.

"Oh, you mean chills?" I observe.

"Yes," he says. "Chills, but much more severe."

Alan doesn't like the fact that he has to take another drug. I see the worried look on his face. I know instinctively that he needs a distraction, so I leave the room to find Michael, Alan's nurse that evening. I find him at the nursing station and ask if he will do the honors of shaving Alan's head. Without hesitation, he agrees. "Just let me find Denny, one of our personal care assistants."

A short while later, the two men come into Alan's room with cutting shears in hand. After much kidding, the ceremony begins. I capture it all on videotape.

When the two men are finished cutting, Denny gives Alan's newly exposed head a buff in shoeshine fashion. We all laugh. It helps ease the tension. Alan looks at me with apprehension and says, "So, how do I look?"

"In all honesty," I reply without hesitation, "you look handsome."

Alan asks for a mirror and I quickly find him one in my purse. When he looks at his reflection, I can see he is not sure who is looking back at him. All I see is an athlete in training. I wonder who he sees.

Soon, the anti-fungal treatment begins. Five hours into it, there are still no side effects, so I feel more assured. But just as I am easing back into the lounge chair next to Alan's bed, he says he's feeling cold. I reach for a blanket in the closet. As I turn around, Alan is shaking uncontrollably. With chattering teeth and alarm in his voice he says, "Rrrrigors."

That instant, I throw myself on top of him and press the intercom button.

"Rigors in room 86!" I scream.

Within seconds, Michael is at the bedside. He calls for warm blankets and Demerol. I continue to straddle Alan's back, hoping to anchor his body. It's all I can do as it shakes out of control.

4th Tool for *Caregivers*
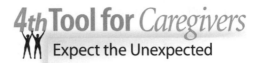
Expect the Unexpected

When the first layer of warm blankets arrives, I hop off and quickly tuck them around Alan. Michael administers the Demerol. It swiftly takes effect and after a few minutes, Alan is still again.

For the first time, I see Alan as a cancer patient. He is tired, pale and bald. It pains me to see him lying there. I kiss him and momentarily turn away.

This is hard.

Not all our moments are low. There are some high points too.

A few weeks later, Dr. Poon enters the room with his usual smile and determined look. I quickly pick up my notepad and pen as he begins to enlighten us about the donor process. We will need to have special blood tests done to determine whether Alan has a suitable donor for his adult blood stem cell transplant. The most likely place to find a match is within Alan's family with one of his three brothers. All humans inherit half of their genetic make-up from their mother and half from their father. The chance of a patient's and sibling's genes matching is twenty-five percent. That means there is a seventy-five percent chance that Alan will not find a match in his family. This doesn't sound very good to me.

I mention to Dr. Poon that Alan has a twin brother and ask if that improves Alan's chances of a match. He explains that a fraternal twin doesn't have any greater chance of matching than any other sibling.

"Then I'd like to be tested as well," I insist.

In his usual forthright way, Dr. Poon replies, "First we'll look at Alan's brothers. Then we'll look at unrelated donors."

"Okay," I say, "but if one of Alan's brothers isn't a match, I still want to be tested."

Dr. Poon nods in agreement as much to appease me as to acknowledge my wish.

Other friends and relatives offer to be tested as well. I begin to make a list of names just in case.

Several of the other survivors on the ward are at the same point in their journey as we are. They too are waiting to know if they have a match and can move to transplant. With the current small size of the average family, only about thirty percent of patients will find a sibling donor. Somehow, I feel we have a slight advantage and I feel guilty for thinking that way. I hold my breath at night thinking of the possibilities.

What if we don't find a match?

I have to tell myself, "Slow down, Cecilia. One step at a time."

Even with their busy schedules, Alan's brothers quickly arrange to be tested. Then, we wait. I find it difficult. We continue with chemotherapy but we cannot move beyond that until we know if we have a donor.

A week passes. I phone Dr. Poon's office to see if there are any results, but there is still no word. That day, Alan has a premonition that Eric is a match. I ask him why he believes this and he says it's just a feeling. I think it will be Alan's twin brother, James, but I keep that to myself. It will certainly make things a lot simpler if Eric is a match since he also lives in Calgary. James lives in eastern Canada and Alan's eldest brother, Dan, lives on the west coast.

On Tuesday morning, I receive a voice message at the hospital from Dr. Poon's assistant, Christine, to call right away.

"I have some good news," she declares. "We have a match."

"Who is it?" I blurt, my heart pounding in my ear.

"It's Eric," she says.

My first thought is, "Oh my gosh, Alan was right. This is great news."

I rush to tell him. When I do, his eyes fill with joyful tears. He immediately calls Eric and leaves him a message. We vow to celebrate together soon. Others on the ward are not so lucky, and I find it hard to share our news with them. Although they are happy for us, I can see the pain in their eyes. They are still searching for that life-saving match.

As the donor, Eric must go through a series of injections of a drug called NEUPOGEN to stimulate the growth of his adult blood stem cells. He takes this on as if he is training for an Olympic gold medal. How fantastic it is to have a brother so willing to do anything for you. I find myself wishing I had had a sister who would have been so devoted and giving to me.

Eric's personality is much different from Alan's. He is constantly joking and his laugh is contagious. Although he's a successful businessman, he knows how to relax and have fun. Perhaps Alan will acquire some of Eric's lightheartedness through the transplant. I can only hope.

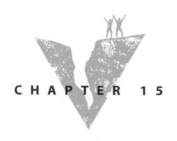

CHAPTER 15

Alan

CAMP

4

"For it is the ultimate wisdom of the mountains that man is never so much a man as when he is striving for what is beyond his grasp and that there is no battle worth the winning save that against his own ignorance and fear."

– James Ramsey Ullman,
Writer, Actor

The moment we received word that Eric was a match, a complex series of events began to unfold that involved hundreds of people. They came from hospital departments of which we had never heard. Many were professionals whose faces we would never see. They worked in tissue typing, flow cytometry (the measurement of cells), apheresis (blood cell collection), the blood bank, radiation oncology, molecular analysis and on and on. Virtually every department in the hospital was involved, from cardiology to psychology, dentistry to pulmonology. The complex coordination of these myriad pieces occurred behind the scenes, largely unknown to me. I marveled at the design of the unbroken chain. If even one of these people had not done his or her job, this page would be blank and our story would not exist.

Over the next several months, we were not only witness to, but wide-eyed participants in a modern medical miracle. Decades of painstaking research by thousands of people, millions of hours of study and experimentation, innumerable clinical trials by pharmaceutical companies, endless treatment protocol tests and billions of dollars in expenditures for everything from blood analyzing equipment to anti-rejection medicines were about to culminate in one overriding and all-encompassing mission – to save a life.

Strangers would soon know more about the microscopic, chemical and biological makeup of my body than I could ever imagine, let alone understand. I was being groomed for an organ transplant except that in my case, the organ was not something you could poke, prod or point out on an anatomy chart. It was my liquid blood, all one and a half gallons of it and, more to the point, the bone marrow from which the blood would be produced.

The sophistication of the process was astonishing. How do you transplant something as inaccessible as bone marrow? How do you interchange a substance buried deep inside something as solid as hardwood? You cannot just remove the defective bone because the affected organ is inside all the bones. Blood cancers are therefore referred to as "liquid tumors" – an unsettling description that implies your whole body is tumorous, which of course it is not. There is no lump, mass or growth. In the case of leukemia, there is only an unbridled release of immature white blood cells into the bloodstream.

The first step in transplanting someone's blood in the treatment of leukemia is to put the cancer into remission using chemotherapy. Although this is not always possible, it is best. The second step, called "conditioning," is to suppress the immune system so it does not reject the new bone marrow that will be introduced. Conditioning not only suppresses the immune system, it also destroys the old marrow. The third step is to replace the dead marrow with new marrow from a matched donor or with adult blood stem cells from which new marrow can develop.

The process of finding an adult blood stem cell donor match for me or anyone in need of a blood or bone marrow transplant is complex. Each of my three brothers – Dan, Eric and James – had a preliminary blood test to analyze his genes. Because Eric's were found to be similar to mine, a long series of more in-depth tests ensued to meticulously compare our respective DNA. Four pairs of genes (hence the eight parameters) were examined. When they all matched and it was determined there were no diseases present in Eric's blood, the transplant was given the go-ahead.

The odds of all this happening, as it turns out, were small. The chance of each of my brothers being a match for me was only one in four. If Eric had not been a full match, a transplant might still proceed depending on how close the match was. If it was not close enough, the search for an unrelated donor would begin through the International Bone Marrow Transplant Registry. The odds of finding a match would then plummet to one in tens of thousands because the donor would not have the same parents as I and thus genetically, our cells would be very different. However, if a partial match was deemed close enough, the transplant might still continue. It was better to die trying than to die not trying at all.

It now became absolutely clear to me why donating blood and getting registered on the International Bone Marrow Transplant Registry were so vitally important. Most bone marrow transplants today are actually adult blood stem cell transplants that are usually painless to the donor. They do not involve extracting marrow from the donor's bones. Instead, the donor simply makes a routine, albeit longer, blood donation over a few hours.

The intricacies of the transplant game became more obvious as we asked more questions. Even with a fully-matched sibling donor such as Eric, the risks remained high. His incoming stem cells (called the "Graft") might recognize my cells (the "Host") as foreign and attack them. A nasty little fisticuff called "Graft Versus Host Disease" (GVHD) could ensue and kill me long before my leukemia did. If I did survive the initial skirmish, my body might still not be able to manage the side effects of this cellular struggle longer-term and I could die from complications of GVHD in the months or years after the transplant. Any way you looked at it, a transplant was a crap shoot. Much of its success depended on medical expertise and equipment. Just as much seemed to depend on blind luck.

But that potential gamble was all in the future – if I had one. First we had to put my cancer into remission. If the cancer was not in remission at the time of the transplant and sometimes even if it was, the leukemia could still come back at a later date and start doing its terrible work all over again. A leukemia patient's best chance of survival lies in putting the cancer rapidly into remission using as few rounds of chemotherapy as possible, then completely killing his defective old bone marrow and quickly introducing the donor's adult blood stem cells. If they engraft quickly and easily, the resulting new marrow produces adult white blood cells that recognize any leukemic cells still lurking around after chemotherapy and destroys them. This is called the "Graft Versus Leukemic" (GVL) effect. It is an important component of achieving a cure using an adult blood stem cell transplant.

The day after getting the news about Eric, I trained for forty-five minutes on the stationary bike on the ward. My hemoglobin was extremely low, but I did not care. The last twenty-four hours had given me renewed hope. When Dale Ens and his daughter, Georgia, showed up with water guns and proceeded to pick a fight with me the next day, the picture was complete. It was strong medicine and I drank in every drop of love they squeezed at me.

A few days later, my blood cell counts hit bottom and began the climb back. Labor Day came and went without much sense of occasion, but Cecilia and I did manage a slow restful bike ride through town along the banks of the Bow River. The rest of our days were spent at the hospital.

One morning during rounds, more daylight broke through when one of my hematologists, Dr. Ben Ruether, walked into my room. He took one look at my blood cell counts and vital signs and said, "We're going to get you out of here today!" Three weeks after being admitted, I was officially discharged from the hospital after my first round of chemo. After a little training on how to keep my central line clean and strict instructions not to immerse myself in water over chest deep (although showers were fine), Cecilia and I set our sights on the next objective – preparing for my second wave of chemo by regaining as much of my health as possible. I rested at home, received wonderful acupuncture and Reiki sessions from Patti Mayer, Jane Stewart and Mary Tidlund, and steeled myself for the challenge ahead.

During this time, I took another important step forward. With head shaven and heart pounding with apprehension, I walked into my fitness club, passed my membership card in front of the automatic scanner and headed inside. To my amazement, the receptionist, whom I had known for years, did not even recognize me without hair. I entered as a stranger.

Chuckling to myself at how little my fears of rejection had materialized and how I had wasted so much time and energy fearfully anticipating a non-event, I got changed and made my way to the fitness floor.

But no sooner had I climbed onto one of the machines than I was instantly recognized.

"Hobson!" a fellow member bellowed to me loudly. "Whatcha do? Get your head shaved for scuba diving?"

"No," I replied, trying to summon up some courage. "I had it chemically removed."

"Whatcha mean?" he bantered. "You shampooed with Neet?"

"No," I quivered, pausing at the edge, "…chemotherapy."

His face fell. For a moment he was speechless. Quickly, he came over to me.

"Oh," he said, crestfallen. "I'm so sorry. I didn't know."

"And there's no way you could have," I replied, trying to give him solace. "The bad news is that a month ago I was diagnosed with acute leukemia and I've recently finished my first round of chemotherapy. The good news is that my brother, Eric, has been found to be a match for a potential adult blood stem cell transplant and things are looking optimistic at the moment."

There was another long pause.

"I don't get it," he queried. "You're such a healthy guy and you're very physically active. How could you get cancer?"

"Anyone can get cancer," I explained. "It's just there."

"You mean like Everest?" he quipped.

"Yeah," I agreed, smiling, "something like that. Actually, it's been a lot like Everest, only harder."

"That doesn't surprise me," he acknowledged. "I've never had it but I know others who have. It's tough stuff. But if anyone can beat it, you can."

"Thank you," I replied. "I'm not sure any of us can 'beat' anything, especially cancer. The best we can hope for is to keep flowing along."

He nodded reassuringly and then gently put his hand on mine. It felt good to know he cared.

The world is simultaneously a kind and cruel place. Where I had feared rejection and ridicule, I found compassion and understanding. The key seemed to be able to find the courage to baldly walk into a public place and say, "I have cancer." No one could help me if they did not know, and once they did, I was usually amazed at the reaction. I discovered cancer survivors everywhere, and that was the biggest boost to my spirits. "If they can do it," I thought, "maybe I can too."

Some people do not know how to react to a cancer patient. They do not know what to say or how to be comforting. The sight of a pale-faced, shiny-domed and sometimes gaunt-looking figure conjures up visions of POW's and victims of famine. It can be frightening, and even more so if it is someone they know or love.

I found that I responded best when people gently asked questions about how treatment was going and listened quietly and carefully to my reply. Telling me stories about others they had known who had died of cancer or the ravages of cancer treatment were quite unsettling. So were statements like, "Hey, you look good," when I knew full well I did not and, "I know what you're going through," when it was impossible that they could. I found "I'll keep you in my prayers" particularly difficult because, although touching and certainly well-meaning, it seemed a little morbid. It was as if they thought I was dying and all I had left were prayers. Heck, I was doing everything in my power to stay alive and I had no intention of dying if I had any say in the matter. Besides, with the help of Raja Yoga, I was connecting with a Higher Power daily, although it certainly could not hurt to have others doing the same in their own way.

My best friends just treated me like me. They talked and laughed with me. A few cried, but not many, at least not when I could see it. Amid the uncertainty of treatment, a little normalcy like pleasant conversation was a welcome change. It was okay to talk about cancer just as long as that was not the only thing we talked about. I really enjoyed getting news about their lives and the outside world because it was something beyond my hospital experience – it was on the other side of the quarter-inch mile.

What really helped spur me on was when someone said that they had seen something in my character that encouraged them. While my body may not have been what I wanted it to be, I knew that if my character was strong, it could not be changed by cancer. The disease could take my body, but it could not take my soul. It could not rob me of who I was. I told Cecilia one day that if I survived, I wanted to become a master – like some of the ancient Chinese teachers or Buddhist monks I had met around Everest. They were masters of their minds.

"Going public" about my illness was difficult – *really* difficult. I did not announce it to the world. I just showed up. Some people thought I had shaved my head to "be cool," and I was grateful I was not a woman who had to grapple with so many more societal stigmas. I could not imagine what it was like for a woman to have her femininity violated by breast cancer and her body permanently altered by a mastectomy. At least I could easily escape detection with a bald head as long as I maintained my weight and muscle mass. A woman had it harder. Each day brought new learning for me.

One day in the apartment elevator, a woman gestured to my head and remarked: "Are you in training?"

"Yup," I answered proudly, "I'm in training for life."

She looked puzzled for a moment and then added: "I guess we all are."

There were other reactions, some surprising. When he learned of my illness, an acquaintance in our apartment building, a smoker, remarked: "Well, if someone as fit as you can get cancer, I might just as well keep right on smoking."

I was amazed at how critically important our attitudes were to our outcomes in life. My belief that cancer could happen to anyone, but that certain lifestyles and behaviors could attract it, seemed to be lost on him. I learned again that we see the world not as it is, but as we are, and that our choices can determine our sorrows as well as our blessings in life. I hoped he would not find that out the hard way and pay the ultimate price.

The price we paid for those days in late August between the first and second round of chemo was long hours of monotony. Time passed slowly, almost interminably. Cecilia and I were satisfied that we had somehow made it this far through treatment, but much as we tried to live in the moment, we were still apprehensive about what lay ahead. So much of the challenge, it seemed, was managing the grinding uncertainty. Cecilia seemed to be better at this than I was. I wanted treatment to be over quickly, but that was impossible. I had to learn to make haste slowly.

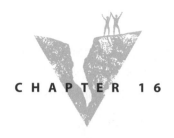

CHAPTER 16

Cecilia
THE STAIRWELL OF MY MIND

Each morning when I arrive at the hospital, I go to the cafeteria to have a multi-grain bagel with cream cheese and a cup of tea. This is becoming my ritual. Then, with my backpack and cooler full of food, I apprehensively approach the stairwell of the Special Services Building.

I take a deep breath before opening the stairwell door, like I'm taking my last breath of fresh air before diving into a bottomless ocean. Some days, I feel like I'm on the ocean floor under thousands of pounds of pressure from the water above.

I force myself to take the stairs rather than the elevator. It gives me a chance to focus on my steps, one at a time. Unit 57 is on the fifth floor. The stairwell is dull and a bit dark. I can hear my footsteps echo through the passage. There are twenty steps between each floor. I count them as I make my way up. Sometimes, a nurse or doctor passes me. I feel that I am moving so slowly. Most of the time, I'm alone with my thoughts. Some mornings, it's all I can do to place one foot in front of the other, but I always continue the climb.

Each morning without fail, I stop in front of the door to the unit, close my eyes and take another deep breath. I hold a happy image in my mind. Sometimes it comes quickly, at other times it takes several minutes to conjure up a picture.

One happy image that comes easily is Alan and I eating sweet juicy watermelon on the fresh green grass outside the hospital. It had been a sunny summer's day, and summer to me means picnics with watermelon. I desperately wanted a sense of normalcy and I was determined we would have a picnic. It might not be on a mountaintop, but it would be outside and that's all that mattered. That morning, along with the regular food for Alan's meals, I packed a blanket and some nicely cut pieces of watermelon. Our picnic was heavenly. Time and again, I would draw upon this image and taste the sweetness of summer in my mind.

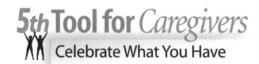

5th Tool for *Caregivers*
Celebrate What You Have

There are other moments I call upon too. One is of my black Labrador, Penny, my childhood pet. As an only child, I did not have any siblings to confide in or play with; Penny was my sister, my best friend and my most trusted companion, ever ready for whatever game I dreamed up. She served as my four-footed therapist, the one who knew my darkest secrets and never judged me. Penny was the first of several dogs with whom I shared my life, although it has been a while since I have enjoyed the friendship of a pet.

Unexpectedly, dogs come back into my life via Unit 57. Alan has been feeling a little low and Rita has an idea. She tells me she will bring her three dogs into town and pay him a visit. I think this is an incredibly generous offer since she will have to bathe each dog before they arrive. Then she'll have to drive from her country acreage all the way back into the city on her day off.

This morning, I bring Alan his usual array of breakfast items, but he doesn't feel like eating any of them. I had planned to keep Rita's visit a surprise, but when I see the sadness in Alan's eyes, I decide it's best to tell him right away. Immediately, his eyes light up – there's a look of anticipation in them.

The cloudless sky seems to promise hope, openness and freedom. The anticipation of an outing has us giddy at the thought of playing outdoors. We meet Rita; her husband, Brian; their son Garret; and their three dogs – Chico, Buster and Oreo – at a nearby green space. It's love at first sight.

Buster is a beautiful Golden Retriever. As I bury my face in his luxurious coat, his soft fur tickling my nose, the anxiety and fear that had been with me when I'd brought Alan his breakfast that morning vanishes.

Alan kneels down in the soft green grass and holds his glove-covered hands up to Oreo, a black Cocker Spaniel with poor eyesight. His hands need to be covered to reduce the chance of contracting an infection. Garret sits down beside Oreo and the three of them engage in a sharing of souls. While Oreo's vision is poor, her other senses are acute. She feels the emotions of the moment – joy, pain and fear. She allows Alan to caress her thick black coat and they both smile at the pleasurable sensation. Garret's boyish laugh has us all feeling carefree again. My eyes fill with happy tears at such a display of emotion. It is as if Oreo knows Alan needs her love, and she gives it openly. I watch with a smile on my face and a glow in my heart as a bond forms between dog and man that transcends most human connections. Alan hadn't felt like eating a thing for breakfast, but after his dog encounter, he has a fruit smoothie and a full dinner that evening. I am overjoyed at this transformation.

"Cancer is a disease of emotion," says Dr. Greg Ogilvie, a veterinarian. "It's a disease of shadows and hallways – the shadows of all the people you've known who died of it, your relatives and friends." I feel the truth of these words. One aspect of the powerful healing ability of pets is their capacity to make the atmosphere safe for emotions. I've known that all my life. Animals are incredible healers.

A few days later, I am again walking toward the base of the stairwell when I bump into three girls coming out of an elevator. Each of them has a beautiful dog in tow. I am so stunned by their presence in such a sterile environment that I blurt out, "What are *you* doing here?" One says she is volunteering for the hospital's animal-assisted therapy program. Intrigued with the idea that there is a formal program for this sort of emotional therapy, I drill her with questions.

One of the girls explains how she brings her dog in once a month to visit patients. They spend an hour and a half at the hospital while patients interact with the happy loving bundles of fur. She says she isn't sure who enjoys the visits more – the patients, the dog or herself. I know I need to bring this kind of therapy to others. I vow that when Alan comes out of the hospital for good (it is never "if" for me), I will volunteer for the animal-assisted therapy program myself. The only problem is, I don't yet have a pet. So, as I make my way up to the ward, I dream of having one.

When I get up to the ward, I peer through the narrow window cut into the door. I push the door open with a smile on my face and the comforting thought of dogs on my mind. Then I walk down the hall to Alan's room.

No matter how difficult the night, no matter how filled with unease, I leave my fearful feelings in the stairwell. Whether it's the image of watermelon or dogs, I try to take only joy into the room.

CHAPTER 17

Alan

CAMP
5

"In a race like this, if you're really good from the shoulders up, you can keep plodding on."

– Mr. Laurie Dexter,
Ultra-Marathon Runner,
One Step Beyond

On September 1, our picture got even brighter.

I came home to the apartment one afternoon and suddenly found Cecilia draped over me like a warm blanket.

"The hospital just called," she said as tears of jubilation ran down her face. "Your latest biopsy shows the leukemia is in remission!"

I felt a surge of energy. It could not be true. It could not be. Not this fast. Not after just one round of chemo.

It was. For a few days, there was even talk about skipping the second wave of chemotherapy and going straight to transplant, but unfortunately the many pieces of the transplant process were not yet in place. So Dr. Poon made a very wise strategic move. He decided that once my blood cell counts had rebounded after the first wave of chemo, he would re-admit me for a shorter but nonetheless substantial wave of continuous chemotherapy.

While we were ahead in the race, he theorized, we would widen the gap.

Buoyed by the news of my remission, Patti Mayer arranged for me to see Dr. Steven Aung, one of a small number of physicians who practice integrative medicine. This combines complementary therapies such as acupuncture, herbal remedies and other ancient healing arts with western medical techniques. Cecilia drove me three hours north to Edmonton where I met Dr. Aung at his downtown clinic.

After a Traditional Chinese Medical (TCM) examination that included non-invasive tongue, pulse, ear and hand diagnostic techniques, I was astonished when he was able to tell me my body temperature and approximate blood cell counts. He also told me how he perceived the chemotherapy was affecting my immune system, which in the TCM system involves Qi (vital energy) and Shen (your total spiritual and constitutional vitality). After an acupuncture therapy session to help boost my immune system, he told me I would rebound from leukemia and the side effects of chemotherapy: "You are like one of those Daruma dolls," he proclaimed. Popular in Japan, these dolls are weighted at the base so that they can never be knocked down, showing that success can follow misfortune if we never give up. "You will recover from this, my dear," he concluded.

All of Dr. Aung's actions, from the tone of his speech to his fluid, measured movements in the room were performed in a deeply contemplative and tranquil manner. I emerged with a feeling of settled disbelief. The skeptic in me went into immediate denial, but the idealist pondered the possibilities. Clearly, Dr. Aung had a vast depth of knowledge and experience as well as an inner peace and harmony. He was a master.

Armed with several powerful Chinese herbs Dr. Aung prescribed to help boost my immune system, Cecilia and I returned to Calgary with a wider perspective on complementary and integrative medicine, especially TCM and its intriguing diagnostic techniques. It seemed like magic, but obviously its methods had passed the test of time – centuries of it. I longed to learn and experience more.

A few days later, I was invited to the memorial service of a friend who had died of uterine cancer. She had been married to a man with whom I had written my third book and I had known the couple for almost ten years. As part of the ceremony, the funeral party climbed a small hill behind what had been their family home in the foothills of the Canadian Rockies. With the mountains looming before us on the horizon, we each took a turn scattering her ashes into the wind. It was a glorious day, but a sad occasion and it caused me to reflect on my cancer journey so far.

That night I wrote in my diary: "I don't want to go over the edge. I don't want to go there – not yet, not for quite a while yet."

On September 25, Cecilia and I were back at the hospital to begin the second "juice festival," and the eternal room swap started again.

Cecilia and I nicknamed my first roommate "Superman." Rod Barnes had worked as a night warehouseman with a large national dairy until he had come down with acute lymphoblastic leukemia (another form of leukemia in which the immature blast cells build up in the lymph nodes) two and a half years earlier. He had somehow survived an incredible thirty-six rounds of intense chemotherapy – not three-hour outpatient sessions, but often a week or more of non-stop infusions. Rod's leukemia went into remission early in his treatment and his adult blood stem cell donor, his sister, had been ready to make a donation. But while doctors debated the pros and cons of a transplant, his leukemia had returned with a vengeance. It had taken him and his wife, Jo Ann, over a year and a half to get back to where they had started. Upon Rod's insistence, doctors had decided to use his sister's adult blood stem cells after all. Now he was only a week away from transplant.

Rod was a shy soft-spoken man of few words. He stood over six feet tall and weighed more than two hundred pounds. His fingers were thick, round and strong, the result no doubt of years spent toting heavy weight around a warehouse. His voice was deep, but muted, and despite his imposing size, he was mild-mannered, kind and peaceful. He chose his words thoughtfully and was careful not to offend. What little he did say had impact, as much because of the pauses that punctuated his words as the words themselves. I liked him right away, and it was not long before he became a friend and mentor. He and Jo Ann had endured unimaginable horrors so far, but Rod was absolutely determined to continue with his treatment. He was going to make it to transplant, period.

"Barnes," I commented one day as we lay in our hospital beds staring light-headedly at the same ceiling tile, "you are one tough guy. How have you survived?"

"Dunno," he reflected. "I just get up every morning. Jo helps me."

In that simple statement, Cecilia and I found substance. We agreed that if we could just keep getting up every morning and mustering a fraction of Rod and Jo Ann's resolve, perhaps the four of us would one day meet again outside the ward. He was slated for transplant about six weeks before me so we looked up to him and Jo Ann as a standard. They showed us that although mountaineers could be tough, a night warehouseman and his wife could be tougher. Rod and Jo Ann were in a league of their own.

A few days later, I was moved to another room. My new roommate was Jim Cleghorn. Twenty-one years old, he had a full face and jet black hair. Rectangular wire-rimmed glasses straddled his nose and a small goatee beard adorned his chin, giving him a bit of a thespian look. He was a keen music fan and a car audio expert, so we talked for hours about everything from stereo equipment to model airplanes. Like me, he had leukemia, but despite a worldwide search, doctors had been unable to find an adult blood stem cell or bone marrow donor for him. As a fallback, nurses had collected some of Jim's own adult blood stem cells. These would be specially conditioned in the hopes that the defective adult blood stem cells could be destroyed. If his leukemia returned after chemo, he would have the option of receiving these "purified" cells back. But if any of them were still diseased, his leukemia could return and he would likely die. His situation was graver than Rod's or mine.

Jim's perspective was different from Rod's. Like me, he hated the confinement of the hospital and wanted nothing more than to escape it as soon as possible. Unlike me, he fought every step of the way. At times he was bitter and angry, and it was easy to see why. His life had barely begun and yet it was in serious danger of ending. At least I had had forty-two years to go after my dreams. He had yet to follow his own dream of starting a car audio business and he was committed to doing so once he got out of the hospital.

Each cancer patient brought his or her own approach to the experience of illness. After rotating through several roommates, however, I began to notice some recurring behaviors. When some patients heard their diagnosis and prognosis, they became deeply depressed and withdrawn. They seemed to fold their tents and give up, convinced the prognosis would become reality and that they would never be able to crawl out of the crevasse. They died quickly. A second group appeared so overwhelmed that they put one hundred percent faith in their doctors and almost completely abdicated involvement in their treatment. They lasted a little longer. A third group was downright angry. Rather than fold their tents, they chose to crawl out and scream at the wind. This was understandable, but in venting their ire (and sometimes suppressing it), they seemed to squander vital energy at the time they most needed to conserve it. A final group, of which Rod, Jim and I were part, experienced all these reactions but ultimately resolved to pack up our tents as quickly as possible and return to what we considered to be our life purpose. That was our overriding mission. Rod wanted to live for his wife, children and grandchildren. Jim wanted to live to be an independent entrepreneur. I wanted to live to inspire others. Cecilia and I would do it together.

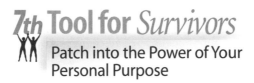

7th Tool for *Survivors*
Patch into the Power of Your Personal Purpose

Nevertheless, it was also obvious that even with a powerful sense of personal purpose, a survivor could not always overcome a disease too far advanced. Attitude was important, but random timing appeared equally so.

I will not speak much more about treatment. Everyone knows it is unpleasant. Through past experience and good fortune, I was able to survive the second wave without infections and essentially without incident. Support poured in from all sides and in ways Cecilia and I could not possibly have imagined. My friend, Linda Brown, an internationally renowned trumpet player, serenaded me with *Dream the Impossible Dream* over the telephone.

After a disheartening day at the fitness club, I realized that in only six weeks of treatment, I had lost half of my strength and endurance. Fortunately, my friend, Hal Kuntze, wasted no time in grounding me.

"Hobson," he expounded, "your goal is not fitness, my friend, it's hemoglobin. You cannot have one without the other, so for the time being you'll have to learn to walk before you can run. The good news is that unlike many patients, at least you can walk. Think what it would be like if you couldn't even crawl out of bed."

One day, Rita and her youngest daughter, Breanne, presented Cecilia and me with a special gift of heart-shaped rocks their family had collected over the course of a decade. They sat at my bedside carefully unwrapping the stones as if they were prized jewels – and they were. Each came with a story of where it had been found, by whom and under what circumstances. This transformed otherwise inanimate objects into precious symbols of the vibrancy of life. Cecilia was moved to tears. Rita and Breanne had chosen to give us a piece of themselves and of their family history. It had far more meaning than any store-bought gift and cemented our belief that the only difference between a rock and a diamond is the size of the person's heart presenting it to you.

Another note of support came from my friend, Carl Hiebert. He had broken his back in a hang gliding accident years before and become a paraplegic, but his love of flight had never left him. I had met Carl in 1988 while traveling across Canada to write the official retrospective book on the Olympic Torch Relay, *Share the Flame*. He had been chosen as an honorary torch bearer in recognition of having made the first flight across Canada in an ultralight aircraft. This "Gift of Wings," as he called it, had allowed him to break free of his wheelchair. He has since become an expert in low altitude aerial photography and specializes in creating unique photographic books that give readers a completely new perspective of the world. By wheeling up to the cockpit of his plane and hauling himself into it, he had given me a whole new perspective not on disability, but ability and courage. He enlightened me by explaining the true meaning of the word FEAR – Future Events Amplified beyond Reality.

One day at the hospital, we received a visit from an energetic woman named Debbie Baylin. She announced herself as a member of the "Art à la Carte" program and showed us a wheeled cart on which were stacked paintings and prints.

"Choose the ones that speak to your spirit," she said buoyantly. "Then we'll hang them anywhere you want."

In no time, Cecilia and I had chosen a few inspirational mountain scenes. These had a surprisingly powerful effect. They helped bring what was outside our window inside our room and served to crystallize the vision of our ultimate goal.

Perhaps my most remarkable experience of that time came during a conversation I had with a farmer whose 18-year-old son, Andrew, was admitted one day with acute leukemia. Andrew had a very serious lung infection and the prognosis looked bleak. I came upon his father, Rae Kopeechuk, seated in 57's sunroom one evening, his eyes downcast and his face pale.

"You look troubled," I observed as I sat down beside him. "What is it?"

"I don't understand," he confided. "I don't know what I could have done to have brought this on. I obviously spent too much time working on the farm and not enough time with my son. I've been a poor friend and a bad father."

"I doubt that," I sympathized. "Life just sometimes has a way of hitting us with some curve balls. Andrew will receive the finest care in the world here. Judging only by his age and the fact that he's otherwise probably an extremely strong and healthy lad, I'd say he stands a much better chance than you or I could know."

"You think so?" Rae asked.

"Absolutely," I affirmed.

There was silence for a moment.

"You seem pretty spry," he finally commented. "Whatcha in for?"

"Acute leukemia," I admitted, smiling as broadly as I could.

Rae looked up at me.

"But you look well. How could that be?"

"They take wonderful care of you here," I said. "And they'll take wonderful care of Andrew too. The best thing you can do for you and your son right now is to stay strong. If he has a lung infection, they'll treat that first. Then as soon as possible, they'll begin chemotherapy to treat the leukemia.

"A crop doesn't grow overnight and cattle take time to fatten. You know that better than anyone else. So hold your ground. It's too early to know if there's going to be a drought or not. One thing's for sure – if your courage dries up, so will his."

His eyes started to well with tears.

"Thank you for lighting a candle in the darkness," he whispered. "You have given me hope."

It did not occur to me then, but Rae and many of the rest of us touched by cancer shared something beyond struggle. We shared blame, especially self-blame. While Doug Rovira had cautioned me against such thoughts, it seemed that blame was another of the many crevasses we could fall into and be incapable of escaping. I grappled with my guilt, as did others, some of whom were not even patients.

The next day, I visited Andrew in his room. It was the same room in which I had begun my treatment, so I related strongly to where he was physically and psychologically. He was a hefty lad, the kind you envisioned in the back forty making his way through a herd of beef cattle as nimbly as some of us pick through traffic. He had broad shoulders, a barrel chest and a thick neck. A tuft of crew-cut, short black hair capped the top of his head. His chin had the hint of a beard.

I knew immediately that Andrew's mind was in the right place because hanging from his television set, written in his own hand, were the words: "I *will* get through this."

Despite his condition, Andrew was conscious and lucid. I admired his drive and determination. His mother, Stephanie, almost never left his side. Throughout his treatment, I checked in with them. He recovered slowly but steadily. When his feet swelled uncomfortably, I loaned him a pair of the fleece boot liners I had used during my training for Everest. Because they were soft and warm, he was able to walk in them and keep his feet cozy at the same time. I smiled to myself when I thought of all the hours I had spent going uphill in them and how they were now helping someone else climb an even bigger peak. Although Andrew had many days of intense discomfort, he never lost hope. We added his name to the list of climbers to see on the outside.

On October 1, Cecilia and I went for a mountain bike ride in the foothills of the Rockies. It was great to breathe in the clean autumn air, to see the trees changing colors and to know that for a few hours at least, we were free. But when Cecilia suddenly tumbled off her bike and landed with a frightening thud, it shook me badly. Fortunately, aside from a bump on her chin and a minor bell-ringing in her ears that left her disoriented for a few minutes, she was all right. Still, the incident brought my life tightly back into focus. I realized, as she had, that my partner could be taken from me at any moment. But while she had not flinched at the prospect of losing me, or at least not shown me her fear, I could not have seen myself being nearly so strong. She set an unmatchable benchmark.

They transplanted Rod Barnes the next day. We sent balloons and I paid him a visit. He was his usual self – steady.

"Well, Rod," I cheered. "Sincerest congratulations! You made it against all odds. I am so proud of you."

"Thanks a lot, Al," he beamed. "It's been a long road."

"You can say that again. I guess there's more ahead, but I just wanted to say you're amazing."

"Not really," he said humbly. "I just lie here and take it."

As I looked on, Rod began to quietly cut the steps and lay the rope ahead of me up the peak. It was so good to watch him begin to crawl out of the crevasse and climb back toward life. He was far from walking off the ward, but he had thrown back the sheets and he was preparing to place his feet on the floor. Whether he would make it to the front door of the hospital we did not know, but we knew that even if he collapsed along the way, he would crawl and when he could crawl no longer, he would pass away, but he would do it on his own terms. He set a standard for me and for everyone on the ward.

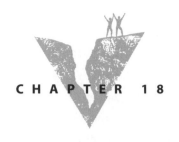

C H A P T E R 1 8

Cecilia
RUNNING FOR
LIFE

Dale says it will be a marathon, but I have never actually run a marathon. I had just started training for a half-marathon when Alan was diagnosed. I do know the strength, determination and pacing that long runs require. I believe I have an understanding of what hitting the wall is like.

I knew from the moment of the diagnosis that this was going to be one long arduous journey. I would have to pace myself. There would be good days and bad days. There would be days I would feel I couldn't go another step. I hoped I would have the stamina to continue. I knew I would have to keep taking the steps one at a time.

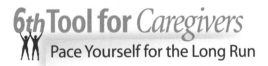

6th Tool for *Caregivers*
Pace Yourself for the Long Run

There are many days when I feel like I am carrying a sixty-pound pack for miles. The pack seems to get heavier and heavier. My shoulders ache from the weight and my feet blister. I feel I will never be able to go the last mile to the finish. There is a point when you say, "I just want to stop here. I can't go another step." That's hitting the wall. You must say to yourself, "I can take just one more step." Place one foot in front of the other and keep moving.

It is October 1, and Calgary is host to the annual breast cancer fundraiser, The CIBC (Canadian Imperial Bank of Commerce) Run for the Cure, a five or ten kilometer walk or run. Standing there in the morning sun amid the hundreds of other walkers, joggers and runners, I proudly wear my Run for the Cure T-shirt. I have written on the back, "I am running for my mother." I look around at the other participants. Some are also running for their mothers. Others are showing their support for a sister, daughter or friend. Many are breast cancer survivors themselves.

My race number flutters in the cool breeze as I prepare for the 10K race. I have no intention of running at the head of the pack. After so much time away from any meaningful exercise, I wonder if I will even finish the race.

It feels good to be outdoors. There is energy in the air and I feel lighthearted and free. I absorb it like a sponge, soaking it up for later use.

Five minutes before the start of the race, my mind jumps to Alan. He is resting after his second round of chemo. The treatments are going well. I trust this trend will continue. I remain positive.

The gun sounds. The serious runners take off, but where I'm standing in the middle of the pack, everyone is at a slow jog – not yet even to the starting line. My lungs fill with the cool morning air. I'm moving comfortably. Slowly, the rhythm of the pack quickens. I am running for my mother, for Alan, and for others touched by cancer.

The run goes well and somehow I make it to the last kilometer. My legs ache. I tell myself this is just a minor inconvenience compared to the pain others have endured during their cancer experience. I repeat to myself, "Mom, this is for you."

Completing the race infuses me with a newfound energy. I find I have enough strength to join Alan on a mountain bike ride in the foothills of the Rockies that afternoon. It is glorious until I fall off my bike and hit the ground hard. My head spins and my world goes upside down.

I get back on my bike and keep riding, just like my mother did and just like Alan is doing. I am determined to finish the race.

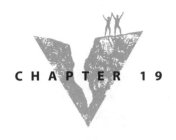

CHAPTER 19

Alan
CAMP
6

"When the situation starts saying: Lose your cool! Pack it in!
Call it quits now! Better go home 'cause now it's going to get
really difficult, that's when something comes up inside me
and says, 'ah, now it's getting interesting!'"

– Mr. Laurie Skreslet,
First Canadian to Climb Mt. Everest,
One Step Beyond

The next day Cecilia and I received a special visit from my former university gymnastics coach, Ken Allen, and his wife, Missy. Ken has been one of the greatest influences in my life. He taught me how to carry on even when I felt weak and tired and how the victory was in the effort, as long as that effort was absolute. We trained four hours a day, six days a week and pushed through fatigue, pain and injuries. And, we had many adventures. We traveled thousands of miles to gymnastics competitions all over the United States by van, mostly with him at the wheel. It was a priceless education, and Ken was an exceptional educator. But his influence extended far beyond the gym. He taught me invaluable lessons about life.

Ken and Missy had come to visit the Canadian Rockies as part of a retirement gift another of Ken's former gymnasts and I had arranged prior to my diagnosis. It was becoming very clear to me how the lessons I had learned in Ken's gym had paid off so handsomely in my cancer journey so far.

"Our attitude at the beginning of a task largely determines our attitude at the end of a task," he once told me.

The next day, after Ken and Missy had left, I would have to put Ken's adage into action when Cecilia, Eric and I were briefed by an oncologist on the risks and rigors of an adult blood stem cell transplant. This was part of a process the medical profession called "informed consent." It involved telling the patient all the terrible things that could possibly result from a procedure ("full disclosure") and then having him sign a form consenting to the treatment. This is as much a legal process as it is a medical one and it forced me to carefully examine my own attitude toward a transplant.

The oncologist assigned to this unenviable task likely had no choice in the process. It was simply his turn in the rotation of routine duties in the transplant clinic. We were horrified to hear that up to fifty percent of patients died within the first year after transplant for a variety of reasons, including failed engraftment and Graft Versus Host Disease, and that there was only a fifty percent chance I would live more than three years after the procedure – if it worked. Even if I did survive, he went on to explain, there was an eighty percent chance I would experience serious chronic fatigue. I could also suffer substantial bone density loss and perhaps even joint destruction because of the powerful steroids I would likely receive after the transplant. If this destruction happened in my hips or legs, I might be unable to walk. Furthermore, what we had understood to be the "cure" that an adult blood stem cell transplant might provide, was actually what the medical profession called "long-term disease-free survival." If the patient was cancer-free and breathing, but incapable of getting out of bed because of debilitating fatigue or joint loss, technically, medically and statistically they were still "cured." The oncologist referred to this state of being as "morbidity," or low quality of life. To me, it sounded like a living death.

This news hit us hard. Whatever hope Cecilia and I had built up from the understanding that my leukemia was in remission and that Eric was a full match rushed out of us like air expelled from a punctured balloon. I was furious.

What the hell was going on? Why had someone not said something sooner? Were they cowards? Was I a coward? Was this some kind of a cruel joke?

What made the whole experience even more difficult was that when the doctor finished his dissertation of doom, he had nothing positive to add. We were devastated.

"So now that you've succeeded in scaring the hell out of us," I said, trying to make light of the situation, "what's the good news?"

Absolute silence and a poker face was his reply.

"Those are the facts," he reaffirmed. "It's important that you be fully informed about the risks of this procedure."

Then he left the room.

I felt like someone had lobbed a mortar into our camp.

"Well," I said sarcastically after the fragments had settled, "that was encouraging. Does anyone have anything else they'd like to add?"

"Not much," Eric replied ascetically, "except that it's obvious this isn't going to be easy."

"Who ever said it was going to be?" I countered. "I'm half inclined to continue with chemotherapy and take my chances. That way, at least I'll still be dealing with all my own cells. There's no telling how much a transplant could kick the crap out of me. At least now I'm able to function. Who knows what might be left of me after it's done."

"True," Eric acknowledged, "but if you decide to go ahead only with chemo, you'll have to live with the constant fear of a relapse. Would you rather face that?"

"Sounds like I could relapse even with a transplant," I noted. "The fear's never going to go away any more than the skeptics or doomsayers are. It doesn't seem like there's any clear way through this."

There was not, and that was exactly the point. Like most big decisions in life, there were no guarantees. There was no guarantee I would even live beyond Christmas. If I did, I might be so dog tired I would be unable to get out of bed. What kind of a life would that be? I wondered whether death might be better.

Now we had a real dilemma on our hands. What we had thought would be a life-saving procedure suddenly sounded like it might actually be a life-taking one, at least by my definition. Even if I survived, I had no intention of spending the rest of my days sleeping or sleepwalking through life. A transplant now seemed to be a journey into the "Death Zone" above 26,000 feet – the more time my life hung in the balance before Eric's new adult blood stem cells began reproducing, the greater my chances of dying of infection because of low levels of white blood cells or internal bleeding caused by low levels of clot-producing platelets. Low levels of red blood cells would certainly mean anemia and serious fatigue.

A blood transplant requires a controlled kill. It would bring me as close to death as medically possible, and then at the eleventh hour, *if* things worked, I was to be rescued using new adult blood stem cells my body hopefully accepted. If it did not accept them, I was a sitting duck for any little bacteria, virus or fungus that wandered by and settled in. It was a ridge walk of frightening proportions.

Cecilia, Eric and I learned many valuable lessons that day. What the medical profession deemed to be "full disclosure" of the risks of a treatment was actually full disclosure of the negative. It was up to us to find the positive. The trouble was that at the moment of diagnosis or during treatment, a survivor and his support team usually did not have the time, energy or fortitude to go looking for hope. They were frightened – usually half to death. I certainly was. The business of finding hope fell to the survivor and the caregiver together. Sometimes we had to dig deep within ourselves to find it, but bad news had to go in one ear and out the other. It could disappoint us, even depress us to the point of despondency, but we could not allow it to deter us from our dream of a better life – or a dignified and graceful death. I was doing everything in my power to avoid the latter.

Dismal or terminal prognoses, negative survival rates, dark statistics, ugly outcomes and portents of doom had to be balanced with optimism – immediately. We could not afford the luxury of a negative thought no matter how much negativity was surrounding us. If we internalized that negativity, it would create an environment in which cancer could flourish.

There is no such thing as false hope, we concluded. All hope is good hope even if it is only a glimmer. Hope was my single most powerful healing tool because it attracted positive energy. Survivors like me at the edge, who had been diagnosed with potentially terminal conditions, did not need doctors reminding us we could fall, even if it was their professional obligation to do so. We knew we could fall. We needed optimists who could give us a reason to hang on – even if it was only to live long enough to see our next birthday. Bearers of bad news, we decided, could serve a purpose beyond the dissemination of chilling information. They could get us to switch our focus to what we had to do to keep from falling.

So, we decided that if treatment had gone so well so far, there was no reason to think it would not continue to go well. The cup *was* half full.

To this point in my treatment, Cecilia and I had believed the entire medical system behaved the way Dr. Poon had. He had told us both sides of the story – that if we did nothing, I might live a year, and that if we did something, I had a better-than-average chance of at least achieving remission. Given both alternatives, we could make our own decision. That was neither positive nor negative. It was balanced. I had signed a simple consent-to-treatment form prior to the beginning of chemotherapy, but the lead-up to transplant was filled with many more consultative hoops. If chemo had been serious, this was more severe. Chemo could make me sick, but a failed transplant could kill me.

Over the next several weeks, we went in search of hope. We began to interview patients, doctors and nurses about the potential outcomes of a transplant. Cecilia researched and compared the results of clinical studies using straight chemotherapy and no chemotherapy versus an adult blood stem cell transplant. Meanwhile, my fraternal twin brother, James, in eastern

Canada, hopped on the internet and began hours of intense research to see what he could discover.

What emerged weeks later was a huge amount of contradictory information. There was still no clear direction in which to turn and most importantly, little discussion that addressed anything beyond living or dying. If I survived, I wanted to know what quality of life I might realistically expect aside from the gloomy predictions we had heard about debilitating chronic fatigue. I began to feel like a climber lost in the middle of a glacier during a blinding blizzard. Snow was swirling in all directions, but I had no compass to tell me which way to go. The more information came in, the more my thoughts turned in confusion and fear. Even my intuition seemed clouded.

A few facts did eventually emerge. Foregoing chemotherapy quickly proved fatal to most leukemia patients. Those treated with chemo who went into remission and received no further therapy usually saw their leukemia return. But those patients who had an adult blood stem cell transplant had a twenty to thirty percent better chance of survival compared with those who only had chemotherapy. We had to do something – now.

The questions, like the fears, plagued me. What would become of me? What about Cecilia? What about our relationship? And there was guilt. I knew there were others on the ward desperately awaiting a transplant, patients who would give anything to be in my situation, but I still found myself hesitating. Should I go for it, or should I retreat? Should I take that first frightening step or should I just sit there petrified on the edge? My transplant demanded a complete commitment. If I decided to go for it, there would be no turning back. I was either going to move forward toward my fear or back away from it. Laurie Skreslet's words danced in my head: "I know that if I want to keep going higher, to see the ground I've come from in a better light, with a better view, I've got to let go of things in the past and go for new things."

I would have to hand my life over to a group of strangers and say, "Here. You take it. Do with it what you will." To some extent, I was already doing that by consenting to chemotherapy but it was a matter of degree. I could still walk away from chemo, but once they started killing my bone marrow to prepare me for transplant, that could threaten me more than physically. If I survived the transplant, would I be a different person because of it? If so, who would I become?

It was a gut-wrenching decision, by far the most difficult of my life. Once I had relinquished control of my body to someone else, would I not be relinquishing control of myself as well? My body, after all, was *me*, wasn't it? And who exactly was *me*?

The questions went deeper and deeper. Everest had never caused this depth of soul-searching. Everest had taught me a lot about fear, but it had never caused me to question who I was. I was an adventurer. I was a speaker. I was an author. No matter what happened on the mountain, I was still Alan, or at least who I perceived as Alan. Now I was not sure who I was. That was the most frightening realization of all.

One of the unsettling aspects of the decision-making process was the effect it had on my relationship with Cecilia. If one-half of a relationship is not sure who he is, it is hard to expect a whole and healthy relationship. At that moment, ours was neither interdependent nor even co-dependent. I was entirely dependent on her and unable to offer her much of anything in return. The energy only flowed one way. This combined with the rigors of the treatment program to create an extremely difficult situation. We no longer had a life outside the hospital. Our daily existence revolved entirely around antibiotics, chemotherapy cycles, blood transfusions and the thousand and one medications involved in this kind of protocol. Ours was certainly a shared struggle, but that is all it was – a struggle. There were moments of levity, but these were few. We focused on getting me better. I wanted to continue to be a cancer survivor. At the moment, that made Cecilia my primary caregiver. Our relationship was not being re-energized. In fact, cancer and cancer treatment were sucking the life blood right out of it. Both of us could sense that a slow and inexorable drift was occurring, but we were at a loss to know what to do about it. We knew there were psychologists in the hospital who might be able to help, so we began to seek one out.

I remembered my brother, Dan, and what he had gone through. It had been his son, Peter James, who had died of leukemia five days before Christmas thirteen years earlier. His second-born son, Michael, had come down with a similar condition a few years later and had had a successful bone marrow transplant. Somehow, through all this, Dan had managed to keep his job, his health and his marriage to Jane intact. They had gone on to adopt a wonderful little girl, Taryn, and they had raised her and Michael with a conviction that loss could be overcome by love. Their family was solid and stable.

"You should call Dan and talk to him about how he held onto his marriage and how he handled the transplant decision," Cecilia suggested. "He's already been over this ground."

Dan is my eldest brother, six years my senior. He had a degree in mathematics and worked as a manager in computer systems operations and sales for a large telecommunications company on Canada's west coast. Sturdy and vigorous, he was an avid outdoorsman like me, but unlike me, he was also an accomplished hunter. Indeed, almost his entire life outside of work and family revolved around moose, elk, deer, duck and salmon fishing seasons. He was used to being alone with himself and nature and had developed a hardy self-reliance, mental toughness and personal resourcefulness I admired. He was frank and honest. When I asked him for his advice, he came straight to the point.

"I understand how difficult this decision must be for you, Alan. This is really tough stuff. A transplant was never really an option for Peter. Chemo basically killed him. Thankfully, Michael was more fortunate and you know the result. He is alive and well and doing wonderfully.

"I really don't know how Jane and I held our marriage together. I've never really thought about it. We just did. You make it through. You have to. The only other option isn't a solution at all. It just creates another problem.

"Neither you nor I know how a transplant might go anymore than you or I know if we're going to be killed crossing the street tomorrow. We can only do our homework today, make the most informed decision possible, and then have the courage to set our compass and stay the course in the woods. Nature will do what nature will do in the same way that a deer will jump in the direction a deer will jump. I don't care how focused we are in our aim or how meticulous we've been in our preparation, sometimes we hit the mark and sometimes we don't. Once we've decided to squeeze the trigger, looking back is a waste of time. So is second-guessing ourselves after the fact if things don't work out the way we hoped they would. The only real measure of success is knowing that we gave it everything we had on that day, at that moment, in those circumstances. In the end, there is only honor."

> *"The only real measure of success is knowing that*
> *we gave it everything we had on that day,*
> *at that moment, in those circumstances."*
>
> – Dan Hobson

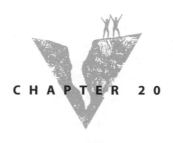

CHAPTER 20

Cecilia
TAKING A
STAND

At an orientation meeting with an oncologist, we learn about the possible long-term side effects of the transplant, one of which is chronic fatigue. To Alan, a life with less than full energy is worse than death. He will not "live" like that, he says. He has always been an athlete, but to me he has always been much more. I believe he has the mental strength and physical ability to be that special survivor who will experience little or no fatigue.

I find myself embroiled in conflict, not with Alan, but with myself. I love him. I want to be with him. I don't want him to leave me like my mother left me more than twenty years ago. So I carefully scrutinize case study after case study on the internet. I speak to doctors and nurses. The results are always the same. The stem cell transplant is the "best" way to "cure" the leukemia. Without it, Alan's chance of survival is slim. I am willing to take the risk, but he's not sure.

At this point, I have to ask myself some very difficult questions. Can I fully support Alan in his decision? If his choice is to treat his leukemia only with chemotherapy, do I honestly believe that this is the best choice and that he can and will live a long and fully active life? If he decides not to go ahead with the transplant and he dies, will the doubts and thoughts of what might have been haunt me? I am afraid to answer these terrifying questions.

Alan is on the telephone with his brother Dan. Dan lost his first son to leukemia; his second son had a bone marrow transplant and has been leukemia-free for years. Alan is expressing his concerns about the transplant and discussing his options. He is telling Dan how difficult the decision is. I can overhear the conversation from the kitchen where I am washing the dishes from our evening meal.

When Alan calls me to the phone saying Dan would like to speak with me, my stomach becomes a ball of fire and my mouth goes dry. I know what question Dan will ask. He knows the tough questions and he asks me the tough question that night. "What do you think Alan should do?" The words are cold and hard, demanding a truthful answer.

I know that once I give voice to my answer, I will not be able to avoid thinking about it any longer. I will know what it is and so will Alan. All my fears will find expression, yet I will also have to take a stand and hold firm to that decision.

With my voice cracking, I say, "Transplant."

"I thought you would say that," Dan replies.

At that moment, I draw my line in the sand. I will now have to defend my opinion to Alan and to myself.

I will not have a restful night's sleep until Alan makes the final decision. I have to be strong.

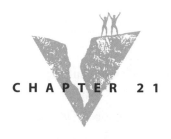

CHAPTER 21

Alan
COMMITTING TO THE
SUMMIT

"Life is such a waste when you're in that confusion
where it's all self-doubt. To hell with that.
Cross the bridge and get moving."

– Mr. Laurie Skreslet,
First Canadian to Climb Mt. Everest,
One Step Beyond

After my conversation with Dan, day by day, week by week, I began leaning towards a transplant. Still, I was not yet fully committed. During that time, Eric received a series of injections of a drug called NEUPOGEN to stimulate the production of the adult stem cells in his blood. On October 6, my mother's birthday, I watched with excitement as he donated what he called his "mother cells." While he joked with the nurses, snacked happily on yogurt and cheese and sipped on apple juice, the buoyant staff of the Apheresis Unit of the Foothills Medical Centre efficiently ran his blood through a centrifuge and separated out about two hundred million of his adult blood stem cells, roughly the volume of a couple of cups of coffee. In six hours, they had collected all they needed. From there, the precious donation went straight into a cryofreezer of liquid nitrogen for preservation at minus 180 degrees [C] until the moment of transplant – if I decided to go ahead with one.

Stem cells are the mothers of all cells. Mature stem cells produce specific types of offspring cells. From adult blood stem cells, for example, come red blood cells, white blood cells, platelets and the many other types of blood cells. Immature stem cells, on the other hand, have no fixed task yet. Called "embryonic stem cells" because they derive from human embryos, they have not yet decided what type of cells they want to be "when they grow up." With scientific intervention, embryonic stem cells may be able to be directed to become any of the over two hundred types of cells in the human body with the exception of the heart. In theory, these new nerve, pancreatic or lung cells (to name just a few) could be used to regenerate damaged, deformed, surgically removed or diseased organs. Embryonic stem cell research may hold the potential of curing spinal cord injury, diabetes, Parkinson's, cancer and many other infirmities. But this type of research is embroiled in controversy. It raises questions about when human life begins and whether the death of embryonic cells during stem cell research constitutes homicide. This ethical debate does not touch an adult blood stem cell transplant for leukemia. No human embryos are involved in adult blood stem cell donation or transplant. The only human who may lose life is the recipient of the transplant if it fails.

When all my cancerous bone marrow had been killed using high dose chemotherapy, Eric's frozen adult blood stem cells would be removed from the cryofreezer, thawed in a small vat of warm water at my bedside and run straight into me via my central I.V. line. The transplant itself, like a typical summit experience on Everest, would take all of twenty minutes, but the patient's preparation for it, just like a climber's preparation for the Himalayas, took months and often years. Living beyond the transplant would be like descending safely from the summit back to base camp. If all went well during the days, weeks and months that followed the procedure, Eric's adult blood stem cells would set up shop in my bones and start manufacturing healthy new bone marrow. This new marrow would then produce brand new blood without blast cells. Voilà, an "instant" oil change – and potentially a new lease on life for me.

Although successful recipients of adult blood stem cell transplants appear to the world to be the same as they did before the transplant, they are very different at the microscopic level. That is because, genetically, anyone who goes through an adult blood stem cell transplant actually has two types of DNA in them. The DNA in their organs is their own, but the DNA in their blood is that of their donor and will remain so for as long as they live. No two human beings have identical DNA and although two types of closely matched DNA can live harmoniously side by side in the same body, they will always be different.

The change from old blood to new, and with it an entirely new immune system created by new disease-fighting white blood cells, would take about three to five years to complete. That was about the same amount of time it took to put together a typical Everest expedition.

When Eric was finished making his donation, Cecilia and I walked with him outside to his car. We each gave him a great big hug. He smiled confidently and said: "There you go, Alan. It's in the bank. Consider it a little life insurance, your ace in the hole. You can play it anytime you want, or not, whatever you decide. I will still love and support you either way. I'm just glad I could be here for you when you needed me."

Despite Eric's commitment to me, the decision about whether or not to proceed with the transplant continued to trouble me. "I don't want to die in fear," I confessed to my friend Dale one day, "but I don't think I'm going to die. I see this just like Everest – big, dark and ominous. Those who go there with arrogance usually don't come back. I just want to go there calmly with as much clarity and conviction as possible. That way, whatever happens, happens, and I can await the outcome in peace knowing we did our homework and carefully weighed all the options.

"When I was interviewing Laurie Skreslet for *One Step Beyond*, he said something about his approach to Everest. He said that it all came down to the question: What are we here for? He was there to give it not just his best, but more than his best – one hundred ten percent, one hundred fifty percent, two hundred percent – every day. Then, even if he failed to make it to the top, there would be no dishonor.

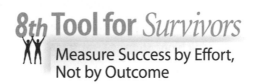

8th Tool for *Survivors*
Measure Success by Effort, Not by Outcome

"I think our situation is very similar, but I'm still not sure whether we should just keep climbing or stand firm and hold our ground," I told Dale.

After weeks of soul-searching, I shared my concerns with Dr. Poon. As usual, he cut straight to the chase: "If you decide not to go ahead with the transplant and elect for more chemotherapy, we'll use the highest possible strength of chemotherapy, several times stronger than what you've already received," he revealed. "The outcomes from a transplant are better than straight chemotherapy and as you've discovered, that margin is about twenty or thirty percent. The best you're going to get with a transplant is a fifty percent chance of survival. No one knows what kind of quality of life you'll have if you do live. So the choice is yours. Is the cup still half full, or has it become half empty?"

Dr. Poon's analysis was the turning point for me. I already knew how chemotherapy made me feel. If I stayed only with chemo, I could reasonably expect to feel significantly worse and I knew what kind of a toll that would take on my body and my mind. It could kill me. If I was lucky enough to survive it, there probably would not be much left of me physically when it was over. I would still have to manage the ongoing fear of a recurrence or relapse, one statistically more likely than after an adult blood stem cell transplant. It was pretty apparent which way I had to go.

The next day Cecilia and I slept in. We arrived at the hospital a little late but at least relaxed. When Dr. Russell came by on his rounds, we announced our decision.

"We're going ahead with the transplant," I said as confidently as I could. "What can we expect?"

Jim peered at me over his bifocals, his forehead furrowing.

"Well, Alan," he explained, "at the very best, the sorest throat you can possibly imagine when we reduce your immune system to near nothing and if you're lucky, a little bit of Graft Versus Host Disease that should take the form of a minor skin rash. At the very worst…"

"We don't care to hear about the very worst, thanks, Jim," I interjected. "We've already been to that movie. The very worst for us is not dying, but ceasing to live."

"I understand," Jim agreed.

"The very worst is not dying, but ceasing to live."

– Alan Hobson

After assuring us he would take the necessary steps to put things formally in motion towards transplant, he bid us good day and left the room.

As soon as he was gone, Cecilia let out a huge sigh.

"What is it, my love?" I asked.

"Thank goodness you decided to go for it," she beamed as a wide smile spread across her face. "I don't know what I would have done if you hadn't. We might have come apart."

"Do you really mean that?" I said, only just beginning to fathom the full meaning of her words.

"Yes, I do," she affirmed, looking flushed with emotion. "I wanted you to make the right decision for you, not for me. Now I can fully support you in it. We're together now. That's all that matters."

I paused to let the enormity of Cecilia's statement sink in. So, I had not been the only one teetering on the edge. She had been hanging out there too, in her own way. As usual, she had not let on. She had just hung on.

I drew her towards me and held her for the longest time, trying to squeeze the tension from her. Together, we looked out the window through the quarter-inch mile. Below, there was a thick layer of fog over the Bow River valley, but as we watched, the cloud gradually burned off with the rising sun. In the distance, two hot air balloons suspended from the heavens made their way towards us, buoyed by a slowly rising mass of warming air from the river below. Surrounded by the window frame, the scene took on the appearance of a picture postcard.

"Isn't it amazing how important perspective is in life?" Cecilia marveled. "From our point of view, there is blue sky above the cloud. But if we were at our apartment downtown right now, we'd only see fog."

We continued to hold each other as the sun streamed in the window. Cecilia was right: so much of life was how we framed our pictures. We could focus on the fog and become lost, or we could tear tenaciously at the cloud until it finally let in the sun to burn the cloud away and lift us above the abyss. Somehow, we had to find the strength to scrape away at the uncertainty enveloping us and then have the patience to wait for the sun to finally appear. Once it did, its rays could penetrate the cold outer exterior of our bodies and warm the inner seat of our souls.

That journey, we were beginning to understand, would take us deeper than a crevasse.

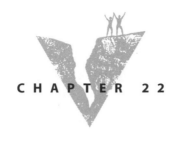

CHAPTER 22

Cecilia
A MOMENT OF DECISION

"The enemy is not cancer. The enemy is fear."

– Dr. Helen MacRae,
Psychologist

Our relationship is strained. The least little thing puts one of us on the defensive. The problem is we don't know what's happening and we don't know why. We decide we need a professional to help us see what we can't see ourselves.

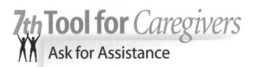

7th Tool for *Caregivers*
Ask for Assistance

Alan and I find a psychologist at the hospital who specializes in working with transplant patients. It takes Dr. Helen MacRae just a few minutes to size up our situation.

I begin by divulging my history with cancer, the passing of my mother and the guilt associated with her departure from my life. Then I go on to give examples of the tension in my relationship with Alan and the unexplained friction between us. Helen listens intently with caring eyes. In a soft comforting voice, she finally says: "Cecilia, you need to do something for yourself every day. At the end of the day, you need to be able to say out loud what you've done for yourself."

I explain that I have tried to stay physically active and do other things for myself, but I just don't seem to have the energy. I've given everything to Alan.

"Then you absolutely must leave something for yourself," she insists, "because if you don't, the worst-case scenario might just occur."

"And what's that?" I ask.

"You don't make it," she replies looking straight at me, "and neither does your relationship."

Alan and I look at each other.

"None of us knows what's going to happen," she continues, "but you both need to know the stakes of this enterprise. They go far beyond one person."

Now it's Alan's turn. He speaks about how he is so dependent on me and how he feels he isn't contributing anything to the relationship. Just like she had with me, Helen absorbs it all. When Alan is finished, she leans forward in her chair. "Alan," she says, "your single biggest obstacle in this whole process is the complete loss of control it's bringing to your life. It's making you feel anxious and afraid, and as a result, you're distancing from Cecilia. She's sensing that and fearing she's also going to get hurt, she's distancing too.

"This experience will take you to a place you have never been to before in your lives. Depending on how you both handle it, you will either grow together as a couple or you will grow apart. As I can see that neither one of you is someone who likes to give up, the choice and the challenge are now yours together.

"The enemy is not cancer. The enemy is fear."

I can see the pain in Alan's eyes. We know she is right.

"I'm now going to ask both of you a very important question," she goes on. "I want you to answer it but I don't want you to say a word. All I want you to do is listen and think very carefully. If your answer to the question is 'yes,' I want you to raise your hand. If your answer is 'no,' I want you to leave your hand where it is.

"Is that clear?"

Alan and I nod affirmatively.

"Okay," she says, "now close your eyes, turn and face each other."

The room goes quiet. My heart is in my mouth. With our eyes closed, there is no way either one of us will know the other's answer. That is scary.

Slowly, Helen speaks: "Are you committed to this relationship?"

My arm shoots up without hesitation. Yes, I am committed. Yes, I want this to work. Then, just as quickly, I feel a sudden twinge in the pit of my stomach. What if Alan's hand isn't raised when I open my eyes? What then?

Helen asks us if we are ready to open our eyes. In unison, we say "Yes."

Our gazes immediately move to the uplifted arm of the other. We embrace one another with tears streaming down our cheeks. We will remain unified.

Inspired by this realization, we leave Helen's office that day hand in hand. We are ready to face the unknown ahead.

At the doorway, I turn to thank Helen for helping us to understand what we are dealing with. "We may need to call on you again," I say.

"I hope you do," she replies. "You guys can do this – together."

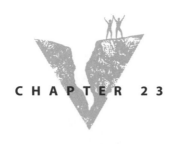

CHAPTER 23

Alan
WAITING FOR WEATHER

"Until one is committed there is hesitancy, the chance to draw back, always ineffectiveness. Concerning all acts of initiative (and creation) there is one elementary truth, the ignorance of which kills countless ideas and splendid plans: that the moment one definitely commits oneself, then Providence moves too. All sorts of things occur to help one that would never otherwise have occurred.
A whole stream of events issues from the decision, raising in one's favor all manner of unforeseen incidents and meetings and material assistance, which no man could have dreamt would have come his way."

– W.H. Murray,
Scottish Mountaineer

Even though our decision had been made, the lead-up to transplant was still a time of continued introspection. On the day after Canadian Thanksgiving I wrote in my diary: "I have a rather gloomy sense of not going anywhere, but quietly marking time." While I hoped to be approaching a renewing life experience, I could not help but think about inmates on death row. Would my decision cost me my life? It was a lonely time, and even though Cecilia was always with me, there was little she could do. We did not have the luxury of seeing anything long-term, much less a potential long-term relationship together.

My body's reaction to treatment presented another challenge. Sudden fevers and infections meant unscheduled diagnostic tests. These added a degree of unpredictability to our lives that left little room for spontaneity. We were willing participants in the process of trying to save my life and understandably, that was our first priority. Given the degree of focus this task required, it was not surprising that our relationship had to take a temporary back seat. Physically, mentally, emotionally and sexually, it was put through a torturous trial. We began to understand how a patient might survive transplant but how a relationship might not. My life and our lives together hung by a thread.

It was a stressful time, not only because of the long-term implications of the impending mega-event, but also because of the shadow it cast upon me. I sought solace in meditation with my spiritual sister, Valerie Simonson, and tried my best to read, although I have never developed it as a regular pastime. My life to that point had been centered around physical activities. With markedly less energy because of the second round of chemotherapy, I found myself lounging around the apartment recovering from the last "juice festival" and waiting for the next conditioning for transplant.

I drew strength from the living stories of those around me. Andrew Kopeechuk was making steady progress. After an hour of preparation, we were finally able to get him outside for five minutes – the first time since he had been admitted weeks before. His energy, determination and vitality were a boost to my spirits. I sensed he would make it.

Rod Barnes was continuing to soldier on as only Rod could, and Jim Cleghorn was his usual staunch self. It was good just to let myself *be* with them and not have to *do* anything. I found great comfort and reassurance in this. It was peaceful. To the other patients, I did not have to be "Mr. Adventurer." I just had to be me. They said I inspired them by walking into their rooms. This was a huge revelation to me. It was almost like being born again, this time without a body, and with only a soul. I sat with them and we chatted about life, death, treatment and dreams. I discovered Andrew had a fascination for Polled Herefords, and although talking about beef cattle was not something I had done much of in the past, I found it pleasant and relaxing. He was a real live cattleman, and unlike so many of his peers, he would likely inherit the family farm and work it himself. That would mean he would have to acquire serious business skills, given the increasing size and complexity of farming operations. That had been the whole reason he had come to Alberta in the first place – to go to agricultural college. He was a tough and enthusiastic young man and I enjoyed his company. He had drive and spirit.

Cecilia used to tease me about spending time with the other survivors. She called me "Dr. Hobson." If the nurses came around looking for me and I was not there, she would just say, "Oh, Dr. Hobson must be out making his rounds," and they would all laugh.

One day I visited a former roommate my age who had the same diagnosis and prognosis. He had stopped eating and he did not look good. I noticed he had few visitors, little family, no significant other and seemed to have lost his passion and purpose for living. His weight was plummeting, so Cecilia and I drove to a nearby ice cream shop and bought him a couple of vanilla and strawberry malts, his favorite flavors.

"Here," I proclaimed, presenting one to him. "Eat this. If you're going to come through this, and you can, you've got to keep your weight up. When I come back tomorrow, I want this to be finished. I'll put the other one in the refrigerator and you can eat it tomorrow."

I was pretty abrupt, but when you are staring death in the face and death is winning, it is no time to play softball. I was worried. He seemed to have lost his desire. I knew that without desire, death could come quickly.

It did. The next day I visited him, he had stopped eating altogether and was in diapers. A few days later, he slipped into a coma and a day or two after that he was gone.

"Damn," I swore to Cecilia as we left the hospital that day. "He could have made it. He could have."

Cecilia put her arm around me.

"Everyone did everything they could," she said.

"I guess he'd just had enough," I allowed.

"I guess he had," she reflected.

As we walked down the hall of the unit, it hit me. The meaning of life is to find meaning in life. Without meaning, there is no life. Is that what had killed my former roommate – a lack of meaning – or had it been leukemia? The pathologist could have told us it was kidney failure or liver failure or whatever. But that was just a symptom, not a cause. I felt the cause was a failure to find purpose, or at least a loss of the will to find that purpose and to see beyond the disease. I had read *Man's Search for Meaning* by Victor Frankl, the psychiatrist and POW in Auschwitz who had somehow survived the horrors of the Nazi death camps. His conclusion after years of unimaginable suffering and intense observation of thousands of emaciated, sick and tortured prisoners had been just that – where there is no meaning, there is no life.

"The meaning of life is to find meaning in life."
– Alan Hobson

In the context of my own life experiences, I knew this to be true. I had either read about it or personally witnessed the power of personal purpose on Everest. At moments when climbers were supposed to perish, when they were freezing cold, exhausted and strung out in the rarefied air, something enabled them to continue. During our first expedition to Everest, I had watched as one of our climbers, John McIsaac, had been caught in a vicious storm. The wind was tearing across the north face of the mountain in gusts of over sixty miles an hour. The temperature was at least fifty degrees below zero and McIsaac discovered that our high camp, his only source of shelter from the fury of the elements, had just been ripped off the mountain. The only thing left of it was a few tattered shreds of tent fabric whipping in the wind.

John had already been climbing for many hours and it was well after dark. Now he faced the ultimate challenge – a nightmarish descent in near hurricane-force wind or death by exposure. It would have been so easy to collapse in the snow, nod off to sleep and never awaken. But that is not what he did.

"Somewhere inside me I found the strength to put one foot in front of the other," he recalled. "I thought of my two little girls, Leanne and Alicia. When I had left my two girls a couple of months earlier, I had promised them I would be back, I would be okay, that I wouldn't die on Mount Everest.

"It was the thought of those two girls in my mind, two girls I love very much, that got me off Everest alive. My two girls are young enough that I was able to use their age as a tool to put one foot in front of the other. I would recall walking six steps and taking a breath, panting for six breaths and saying to myself, okay, that's you, Leanne. I would then visualize Leanne's look as I left the airport. Then I would do the same for my daughter, Alicia, who is nine years old.

"It was that vision, that intensity of love, that got me off Everest."

The day my former roommate died, I went home from the hospital disturbed and afraid. I did not want to die like he had. Although I was going through the motions of life and trying to stay physically active, eat, sleep and drink, I still did not feel alive. The spark was missing. I began to become afraid that I too had lost the spice of life, that even if I regained my health, I might never rediscover my zest for living, my passion for speaking or my relationship with Cecilia. I recalled the moment when I had come across a corpse on Mount Aconcagua in the Andes of South America. A day before, the frozen form had been a brilliant French doctor who had become dehydrated in the cold dry air, developed cerebral edema (water on the brain), collapsed and died. Opportunistic climbers had come by the spot before me and scavenged almost everything of value from his body, including his climbing boots. His rigid remains were wrapped in an emergency blanket slowly shredding in the wind. Only tattered wool socks stuck out on frozen feet from the end of the grisly silver wrapping.

I remember stepping over him, walking about fifty feet further up the mountain and glancing back at his ghastly face. Despite the horror of what I saw, I knew that no one had ever died of cerebral or pulmonary edema without becoming weak from lack of food or dehydrated from lack of water. So I turned my gaze uphill, took a huge gulp of water, sat down and had something to eat. That is what I needed to focus on.

Like then, I now had a choice. I could allow myself to be shattered by the death of my former roommate, or I could use it to sharpen my focus on trying to return to a full life. I had to forget about dying and reconnect with living. It was time to return to the Rockies.

That weekend, my brother Dan, Cecilia and I arranged for a getaway in the mountains. Now that I was off intravenous antibiotics and able to be free of the hospital for at least a few days, we rendezvoused in southern Alberta. We had a wonderful time biking and hiking amid the summits, sharing the starlit nights and sitting in the peaceful silence. I drew power from our surroundings and bathed in the energy of the infinite.

I enjoy a special kinship with Dan, mostly because our personalities are very similar. Dan is an intense fellow. When he goes fishing, he gets up at 4 a.m., and when he goes hunting, he often backpacks high into the alpine wilderness above the tree line, sometimes alone, hoping to catch an unsuspecting deer emerging from the shelter of the forest at dusk. He always hunts on foot, he is deadly accurate with a rifle, and I pity any unsuspecting animal that happens into his sights. Physically fit, highly skilled with a map and compass, and absolutely cunning, to me he epitomizes what a real hunter is. He is a practiced, safety-conscious and ethical outdoorsman with a true love of the hunt and of nature. And, he always packs out what he kills.

While some may argue that any hunter displays a lack of love of nature by killing an animal, the more time I spend with Dan in the woods, the more I come to understand how long and hard he works for a single shot at an animal, how often he is unsuccessful and how much he learns from each new experience. Although I could not bear to dispatch an animal, he and I are alike. He is a consummate adventurer. For Dan, as for me, an outdoor experience might have a stated goal, but it is really just a means with which to explore nature and ourselves. The rules of the game are clear. We are not in control. Nature is. We have to surrender to her. I wished I could approach my cancer experience with such clarity.

At the end of the weekend, Dan returned to work and Cecilia and I continued on to southern Alberta's Waterton Lakes National Park, where we had first scuba dived together on that blustery December day almost four years earlier. I was thankful I still had enough savings and a small monthly disability insurance check so I could afford to focus on re-energizing between treatments and not worry about financial affairs or the demands of a busy family. I knew many survivors were not so lucky, yet those with children had a powerful reason to live.

Our escape to wind-blown Waterton was short-lived. We had been there only a day when a phone call home revealed that Eric's daughter, Laura, had been admitted suddenly to the hospital with a lump in her abdomen the size of a grapefruit. Eric's voice was cracking with emotion. I knew immediately the situation was serious. What a year it had been. First me, now Laura. Was it cancer again?

Cecilia and I drove straight home. It was strange to walk back into the Foothills Medical Centre again, this time not as a patient, but as a visitor. Laura, who was in her mid-teens, was understandably reserved. I tried my best to encourage her, but without success. The mood was decidedly tense.

I gave Eric a hug. I could only imagine what might be going through his mind. Exploratory surgery was scheduled for a few days later. We waited.

It was almost unbearable. Here Cecilia and I were approaching our own critical juncture, and my niece was approaching hers. The good news was she would get her answer sooner than we would. The bad news was it might be worse for her.

When we got home from visiting Laura, I went straight to the gym to blow off steam. I did not have much to blow off and tired quickly. I was dejected. I wondered if Laura would be okay. I wondered if Cecilia and I could make it together. I wondered about so many things. Uncertainty circled like the hands of a clock.

The next day, doctors removed a large cyst from Laura's abdomen. Thank goodness it was benign. Everyone breathed a huge sigh of relief. It seemed cancer had not struck twice in the same family in the same year. I was so grateful she did not have to go through chemo, radiation or more surgery. She would recover quickly and completely.

That week, I began a battery of tests to establish what doctors called my "baselines," or pre-transplant physiological levels. They covered the gamut – eye exam, dental check-up, chest x-ray, bone density scan, even a psychological test. Each was conducted with impressive speed and efficiency.

As we were on our way through the hospital one day to one of these tests, a voice called to us from the cafeteria. We turned and to our amazement saw Andrew Kopeechuk devouring a huge plate of French fries. His intravenous line was gone, he was sporting jeans and a baseball hat, and from all appearances he looked like he could be preparing to head out to feed his cattle. The vitality was back in his voice, as was the twinkle in his eye. He did not look like a cancer patient anymore. He looked like a normal, healthy, eighteen-year-old, ready to take on the world. A rush of adrenalin coursed through us. We congratulated him on getting back on his feet.

A few days later, Cecilia and I reported to the Bone Marrow Transplant Clinic in the Tom Baker Cancer Centre. Only one small but important task remained before transplant. I had to sign the consent form.

A senior nurse, Laura Karlsson, presented me with the document and handed me a pen. She did not say a word. She just looked at me and smiled.

Amazingly, I found myself hesitating. I did not want to sign. I did not want to let go. I did not want to fall.

"Tell me a bit about yourself," I asked her, stalling for time.

"Well," she said, "you may not know this, but I'm good friends with Karen March, the wife of the late Bill March."

"Oh my gosh," I thought to myself. Bill had been the leader of the first Canadian expedition to Everest, the one during which Laurie Skreslet had summited. Like Laurie, Bill had been a hero and mentor to me, a man who had helped spark my Everest dream by taking me on my first expedition to high altitude. I had quite literally climbed in his footsteps on the dormant snow-covered volcanoes of Mexico years earlier and written about him in *One Step Beyond*. Then suddenly, in 1990, he had collapsed on a mountain trail while hiking and died at the scene. Although an autopsy was performed, no cause of death was determined. He left behind a wife and son and a legacy of inspiration, including hundreds of outdoor leadership students he had instructed around the world.

"Bill inspired me to go to Nepal," Laura went on. "I spent two months in Kathmandu while working there towards my nursing degree."

Laura knew Bill would have wanted me to take on this medical mountain and would have been a source of strength for me throughout my climb, regardless of how rough a ride it was. But she understood the sensitivity of my situation and chose to keep those thoughts to herself. She opted instead for a subdued, more professional approach.

"I gather you knew Bill," she commented.

Did I know Bill? Absolutely. More than that, I knew what Bill stood for. He stood for strength, courage and determination. And he stood for hope. When half his team had decided to leave Everest in a storm of controversy, he had stayed to lead the remaining members to victory.

Just then a presence entered the treatment room. It filled the sterile interior with warmth and energy, transforming the cold space into a reassuring sanctuary. I could not miss the message.

"Oh Christ, man," I heard Bill bellow straight into my ear in his unmistakable Essex accent. "Get on with it!"

I signed.

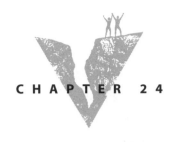

CHAPTER 24

Cecilia
RETREAT

Patti Mayer extends us an invitation to attend a weekend getaway. It is a retreat for couples going through cancer treatment. I am uncertain about attending. I'm afraid it will be a weekend filled with sorrowful faces talking about the drudgeries of their cancer experiences.

Patti explains this is a retreat to re-energize. It will offer Qi Gong (Chinese energy building), Reiki, meditation, calligraphy, native healing and healthy food.

"It sounds interesting but...," I start.

She stops me in mid-sentence. In her soft, reassuring voice she says, "You need this time away." With that, Alan and I agree to go.

My initial concerns about an emotionally draining weekend are dismissed as soon as we arrive. Alan and I drive the fifty or so miles to a wonderful corporate retreat center in the foothills. The cedar log structures with open windows and welcoming entrances help us feel right at home. There is a light dusting of snow on the ground as we make our way from the car to the lodge. Inside, a roaring fire provides the perfect ambience.

One of the retreat facilitators directs us into a smaller room where there are chairs arranged in the shape of a horseshoe. Slowly, couples file in and take their seats. I feel a little apprehensive, not knowing what is expected of me. The facilitator begins by throwing a ball of twine at one of the participants. She asks each individual to say what they are most grateful for in their lives and what they love. Then, while holding onto the twine with one hand, they are to throw the remaining ball to another person in the horseshoe.

I catch the ball and say that I am thankful for the possibility of a second chance and that I love the sunrise in the mountains. Then I throw the ball to Alan. By the time it has been thrown to every person in the room, we have spun a web connecting each of us together.

Next, we venture outside into the cold night air to listen to native music. It takes me away. Much like my Run for the Cure, I become lost in the rhythm. I can feel the sound waves from the beat of the drum reverberating on my chest. It is so natural and primitive. The apprehension I felt earlier is replaced with a comforting heartbeat. I feel I am back in the womb, safe.

The next day, I awake to a brilliant sunrise. We attend a Qi Gong class that starts the day with energy. It involves making sounds and taking deep breaths. The remainder of the morning is filled with all the other activities. When massage is offered from 2 to 4 p.m., I quickly sign up.

Just before lunch, I take a walk around the grounds. To my amazement, I come upon a trampoline. I quickly kick off my shoes and hop on. First I take a little jump, bouncing up just a foot. Then, with more confidence, I try a higher bounce. Now I am reaching for the sky with five feet of air beneath me. I giggle with joy. With each jump, I laugh a little harder. Suddenly, I am a child again.

Soon it is my time for a massage. I lie motionless on the table, trying to relax. I can feel how tight my body is. My vigilance over the last several months has left me tense and rigid. The massage therapist immediately goes to work on my neck muscles. To the taped sound of ocean waves lapping against the shore, I feel her hands slowly rise and fall over my arms. The sweet scent of lavender fills the room.

Within minutes, I feel my body giving way. Before I realize it, there are tears streaming down my face. Slowly, the therapist gently pushes the stress and anxiety from my body. I hear Helen MacRae's voice in my mind, "Do something for yourself each day." Yes, I pledge, I will.

The massage gives me the opportunity to release some of the pain I have been holding inside. I feel warmth and love.

The weekend replenishes my energy, my heart and my soul.

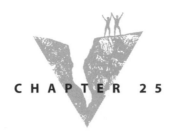

CHAPTER 25

Alan

PREPARING FOR THE SUMMIT BID

*"If you're lucky, once in your life, you come to a place
where you realize you must make manifest
what you profess to believe."*

– Mr. Laurie Skreslet,
First Canadian to Climb Mt. Everest,
One Step Beyond

The last hurdle prior to transplant was another bone marrow biopsy. Dr. Ahsan Chaudry, one of the workhorses of the transplant and oncology program at Foothills, had his work cut out for him. Because of years of training with a heavy backpack, my hip bones were thick and solid. I cheered him on, taunting, "C'mon, Ahsan! Is that all you've got? Torque, man, torque!" He pushed and pulled with everything he had and soon was wiping the sweat from his brow. Cecilia held my hand. It was so reassuring to have her there. Her touch was cool and firm. While all I had to do was focus on the wall and try to stay as relaxed as possible, I wondered how she could keep from fainting. In many ways, I had the easy part.

I am sure Ahsan, the attending nurse and the lab technician were convinced I was a lunatic. There I was, actually encouraging someone to dig into me with a six-inch screw needle. Many patients preferred to be sedated through the procedure. Although I never had the guts to watch what was going on behind my back, I did not fight or resist. I gave in to it. I saw it as another chance to flow. Laughter and cheering were a way to make things easier for everyone. Eventually, Ahsan got what he needed and Cecilia and I went home.

Conditioning for transplant was to begin the following week. To prepare myself mentally, I went up to the ward one last time. I was surprised to see that a transplant survivor, Wayde Gallant, who had received new bone marrow about a month earlier, had not engrafted and had been readmitted with a serious case of pneumonia. His mother, Delia, and his father, Wilfred, had come all the way from the province of Prince Edward Island, on Canada's east coast, to be with him. Wayde's condition reminded me again of the risks I was about to assume. His experience underscored the high probability of infection I would face if Eric's adult blood stem cells did not engraft quickly and I was left without an immune system. In this indeterminate state between the death of my old immune system and the rebirth and reconstruction of my new one, a period of up to three years, almost anything could happen. I hoped Wayde would make it and that both of us might someday be able to celebrate together, perhaps with Rod, Andrew, and Jim Cleghorn on the other side of the abyss.

The high dose chemotherapy that conditioned me for transplant was considerably more intense than the chemo I had experienced earlier in my treatment. I knew they were going to hit me with the big guns when they pre-medicated me with *three* doses of Zofran on the first day and gave me anti-convulsants as well. One of the biggest hitters was a powerful drug called ATG, a hormone derived from rabbits that would make me violently ill. Following Rod's lead, I just lay there and accepted it. I had let go. I knew that somewhere Jim Russell was watching, and that over the years, through trial and error, he and thousands of clinicians like him had developed a progressively more refined method of conducting an adult blood stem cell transplant. That month alone, there would be eight on Unit 57 and over one hundred and fifty in a typical year. That gave me solace. I knew the staff was practiced and I was not alone.

The point of no return came at exactly 8:50 a.m. on November 9. At that time, I began receiving the chemo that would kill my old bone marrow. As the nurse hoisted the bag of clear liquid up on my I.V. pole and released the little plastic valve that would allow the drug to flow through my central line and into my heart, I felt a shudder sweep through me. It was my old foe, fear. But I also sensed that my old friend, Bill March, was there with me, so I let the two of them struggle for supremacy. I had decided long ago to stay out of the fight.

"You can relax," the nurse said as she checked to ensure the chemo was flowing smoothly. "This won't hurt a bit."

Over the next sixty minutes, I said goodbye to my old immune and blood systems.

"How do you feel?" Cecilia asked as she kissed me.

"Anxious," I admitted. "Just anxious."

As I lay in bed, I remembered something the author of *Seven Years in Tibet*, Heinrich Harrer, had once written: "I believe that no man can be completely able to summon all his strength, all his will, all his energy, for the last desperate move, until he is convinced the last bridge is down behind him and that there is nowhere to go but on." That is where I felt I was.

At that moment, the personal care assistant, Bolek Babiarz, walked into my room. He was carrying something we will cherish for the rest of our lives – a cardboard cutout he had made of three "mountains" constructed from discarded boxes. On one end was Mt. Everest, on the other was its sister peak, Mt. Lhotse, and in the middle, the biggest of the three peaks, was my medical mountain. Bolek's creation came complete with rope, anchors, a little photographic cutout of me climbing and even my own miniature base camp tent. He had hand-painted the entire scene in white and blue, pasted the words "CAN/WILL" at the summit of my medical mountain and hand-written a little note along the bottom. It read: *"Consider this another mountain to climb in your life, Alan, so be strong. Never give up my friend.*

Your friend, Bolek."

While we wiped the tears aside, Cecilia and I each gave Bolek a long slow hug. His warmth enveloped us, his kindness overwhelmed. It was the tangible manifestation of something very special, very deep and very strong.

When I had finally collected myself enough for words, I announced: "So let the climb begin!"

"Okay my friend," Bolek replied, gesturing to his creation. "You lead."

For the next few minutes, Bolek and I played like kids. First we glued the tent in place. Then we tied my little figure into the rope and anchored it to the mountain. Together we took turns moving "me" higher and higher up the peak.

"Not to the summit yet, Bolek," I cautioned. "We're still on our way there, pal."

When everything was at last in position, Bolek left. Cecilia and I just sat back on the bed and admired his workmanship. Slowly, I got up and went to the window. On the other side of the quarter-inch mile, it was snowing.

"At last," I observed to Cecilia, "at last it's winter."

"Yes, it is," she agreed. "And spring always follows."

In an hour, the corner had been turned. The nurse came in, detached the spent bag and immediately put up the next one. She told us not to stray too far from the room because she needed to monitor me for side effects. Since I felt quite light-headed, I freely obliged. I just stared up at Bolek's magnificent artistry, held Cecilia close and marveled at the wonder of life.

By mid-afternoon of the second day, I was out on a pass with a portable pump and an even bigger waist pack than before. This one was filled with three-quarters of a gallon of saline solution containing potassium to maintain and replace critically needed water and minerals that would be leached from my body during conditioning.

That evening, my moral support kicked into high gear. My twin brother, James, flew in for the weekend from eastern Canada. He was a tall man, standing six foot one, and had blue eyes and short brown hair. Thanks to regular physical activity, he had a powerful frame, long arms and distinct jaw muscles. My father had always said that James was the nicest of his four boys. He was right.

James was a thoughtful and perceptive man who spoke kindly of everyone. He made his living as a computer consultant and was responsible for helping maintain the software that tracked the Prime Minister's correspondence from the public and generated swift replies. Because Canada's head of government receives thousands of letters and emails each day, it was a task that required around-the-clock vigilance, a methodical mind and above all, a cool head. Even if others screamed at him when the software inexplicably crashed and the correspondence instantly piled up, he had to remain calm and systematically find a solution. This required not only an extensive knowledge of computer hardware and software, but supreme patience and self-control. These assets, perhaps as much as his substantial technical skills, had been some of the keys to his success. My father called him a "brinkman." He was good at the edge.

James and I had always enjoyed a close relationship. Once, as kids, we had conducted a little experiment at summer camp to measure how close we actually were. First, James had shown me five cards he had picked from a deck. Then he had gone to another cabin and thought about one of them for five minutes. When he returned, I had to choose which card he had telepathically "shown" me.

I chose the right card nine out of ten times. Evidently, it is true what they say about twins, at least *this* set of twins. We are linked not only genetically, chemically and biologically, but psychologically as well. Yet oddly enough, James' genes had not matched with mine. They had matched with Dan's.

It was great to see James again. He came bearing gifts – photographs of my niece, Sarah; nephew, David; and sister-in-law, Anne; all specially mounted on foam board, and stories of home. We sat up until midnight talking and then turned in. I slept poorly, having to get up every ninety minutes to pee, thanks to my little three-quarter gallon friend.

At 6:30 a.m., Cecilia and I awoke bleary-eyed. By 8 o'clock, we were all at the hospital. James went everywhere with me. I took great pride in introducing him to everyone, explaining he was seven minutes older and almost seven inches taller. I joked that I had received the recessive gene and that because James had had longer arms as a child, he had gotten to the food faster and outgrown me. Cecilia noticed he was softer spoken than me, but just as meticulous and precise, traits we had inherited from our father. But while James is a settled family man, I am more of a free spirit.

That evening, we drove to Eric's for dinner. I had trouble directing Cecilia to his home, an obvious indication I was not thinking clearly. After half an hour of driving in circles, we finally had to pull into a gas station and ask for directions. I was frustrated and embarrassed to be unable to remember something that before my treatment had been second nature to me. James, sensitive and supportive as always, said nothing. He just went inside and got the information we needed.

"The situation is only temporary," he said reassuringly as we studied a map. "Let's just see where we are."

When we finally got to Eric's, I noticed that something was different that night. I felt removed from the gathering, like I was watching it from the outside. Although I was physically present, my mind was elsewhere. This was the way it would be for me for almost a year after the transplant. It was more than the effects of chemo and conditioning. I was unable to connect with anyone, even at times with Cecilia. I felt isolated and alone. Amid the laughter and cajoling that was as much a part of Eric's home as it had been the one of our upbringing, I could not relate to anyone or anything. The conversations lacked meaning. Everyday comments seemed insignificant.

"Is this really what people think is important?" I thought to myself. "If so, where do I fit in? I used to fit in somewhere, but now I don't feel as though I fit in anywhere. Where do I belong – at the hospital?"

After dinner I went to the living room and lay down on the sofa. Cecilia soon joined me, but there was little she could say or do to reach me. I felt like I was in another world. The magnitude of the cancer experience, coupled with the endless inactivity and sheer monotony of treatment, had worn me down. It was a slow, slow game this one, just as it had been at high altitude – one small step after another and another and another, a little effort, a little rest, a little more effort, a lot more rest. Minutes passed like hours. As the clock ticked toward transplant, I felt like a part of me was dying.

We drove James to the airport the next evening. It was hard to see him go. My twin brother, another precious link to my past, boarded the plane. I watched it take off and disappear into the night sky. Would I ever see him again?

Within days, my genetic proximity to Eric would increase a thousand-fold and we would become closer than brothers. We would become blood brothers. What promise there was in the world and in the universe that in such a time of trial, there could still be the potential for triumph.

It was time for the transplant.

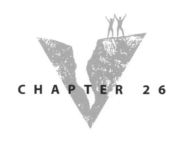

CHAPTER 26

Cecilia
A LITTLE
CONTROL

It is a cool November afternoon and the sun is streaming through the kitchen window, illuminating the room. Our two-bedroom apartment is on the twenty-ninth floor of a high-rise in downtown Calgary. One bedroom is for sleeping and the other is filled with outdoor equipment. Expedition clothing for every season hangs from racks, dotting the white walls with bright colors. Shelves that run from floor to ceiling are filled with gear for any outdoor activity. Skis protrude from behind a bookcase overflowing with maps and trail guides. The ice climbing gear is neatly arranged in an old armoire. Much of Alan's Everest gear is stored in here.

This has been Alan's home for more than ten years. To this point in his life, convenient access to downtown and the airport has far outweighed any need for luxury. He is a guy used to living in a tent. The bare essentials are all that matter. If the heat works, it's a great place to live.

The carpets and upholstery were cleaned earlier in the week by a professional service. Now, with all the plants removed to reduce the risk of fungi in the soil getting into the air, the apartment looks more like a hospital room than a warm inviting home. Today I tackle the kitchen. With toothbrush in hand, I kneel on the cold linoleum floor and begin cleaning the baseboards. My thick rubber gloves make it hard to hold the brush. I dip it into warm soapy water and begin disinfecting the kitchen.

Visions of those damn WASH YOUR HANDS signs keep me focused on the job I must do. I read the entire transplant manual twice, highlighting those areas I deemed most important. The first three sections provided an introduction to leukemia, general information on the transplant experience, the complications and side effects of an adult blood stem cell infusion, what to do while in the hospital (including rules and guidelines for visitors), daily treatment routines and the criteria for discharge.

It is the fourth section in the manual that I am fixated on now, "After Discharge." I have been diligent, perhaps militant, in all areas of Alan's care. I ensure he takes his medications on time, and I wash my hands constantly and remind him to do the same. I limit visitors and minimize the risks of infection whenever possible. I do all these things because they are the only actions I can take. Taking action makes me feel like I am contributing to the success of this endeavor.

I was a naïve teenager when my mother was ill. She didn't talk to me about her cancer and I felt helpless. In the end, she passed away, and I live with regrets of not having done more. I will not have any regrets this time, no matter what the outcome.

One day during Alan's treatment, I was feeling like I was coming down with a cold. I was so angry for allowing myself to become run down. If I have a cold, Alan can't come home and I can't care for him. That evening, I took extra care in the preparation of his dinner, washing my hands constantly, trying not to even breathe in the direction of the food. Before going into his room at the hospital, I stopped at the nursing station to get a surgical mask. I placed the itchy white mask on my face, comforted that it covered my frown. When Alan saw me, he looked puzzled. I explained that I thought I was coming down with something, so I sat on a chair next to his bed without even kissing him.

Even with all my diligent handwashing, vitamin-taking, proper eating (some of the time at least) and going home to sleep a few hours each night, I couldn't avoid getting sick. I wasn't sick like Alan was, but I wasn't in control as much as I would have liked either.

What I didn't realize at the time was that all my efforts to stay in control were just a way to keep fear at bay. Leukemia is a multifaceted disease. I cannot control the outcome of the transplant and it can have numerous complications. I have no control over whether the donor stem cells engraft, or if they attack the host and Alan suffers from Graft Versus Host Disease.

The biggest risk of transplant is infection. Right or wrong, this is what I feel I can have some control over. I will do everything in my power to eliminate this barrier to our success. In my mind, if I can reduce the possibility of infection by keeping the apartment ultra-clean, I can minimize Alan's risk of complications and increase his chance of success.

My need to influence this one aspect is so strong that it outweighs reason. So I am scrubbing the baseboards with a toothbrush. I know this is a bit much. Is it obsessive? Yes. Does it cause tension between us? Yes. Can I say that all my hard work is paying off? I think so.

Alan is alive.

CHAPTER 27

Alan
THE SUMMIT
BID

*"The energy in the room on transplant day is electrifying.
The adrenalin is flowing through my veins as if I am under
attack. In a way I am. There is so much riding on this day, so
many questions to be answered. Is this the right decision?
Will the transplant be successful? Will Alan experience
chronic fatigue? I can feel my pulse quickening and my heart
racing. My face feels flushed and my palms are moist.
I try to think positive thoughts."*

– Cecilia

The day we had been waiting for, November 15, dawned as had every day of the four months since my diagnosis – with hope for the future. This day we would roll the dice and take the ultimate gamble. This day, we would play for all the marbles.

My first visitor was Bolek. He knew what day it was. Although adult blood stem cell transplants were almost as common on Unit 57 as oil changes were in busy service stations, he still was excited. He broke the tension by pulling out a pen, walking up to my daily blood cell count calendar on the wall and creating a delightful drawing of a group of smiling stick-figure adult blood stem cells coming down a ladder. He called them my "Happy Cells" and they filled the entire day on the calendar. Within minutes, he had me feeling happy too.

The last few days had been brutal. I had sometimes been so nauseous, I had been incapable of speaking. When I did retch, it was violent, like something inside me was tearing away. But that morning, miraculously, I felt much better.

"You look good," Bolek said, "considering what you've been through. Today they will try to fix you."

"They can forget it," I said wryly. "My parents have been trying to do that for forty-two years and they haven't succeeded yet. I doubt whether a few hundred million stem cells will even come close to doing the job."

"Well, I guess we'll see about that," he said with a smile.

Cecilia arrived promptly at 8:30 a.m. She was her usual effervescent self, or at least she appeared that way. Whatever she had gone through the night before at home alone – the restlessness and anxiety, the overwhelming need to cry and release all the pent-up tension – she had left there. She knew she had to walk into my room with love and confidence, or the appearance of confidence.

The transplant was scheduled for 2 p.m. Within minutes of my rising, the nurses were pre-medicating me with a heavy dose of sedatives intended to keep me calm and help prevent possible reactions to the stem cells. They had little calming effect. I approached the appointed hour in much the same way I had approached my departure from the South Col at 26,000 feet on summit day. I chatted casually with my colleagues, in this case the nurses, and tried to preserve what little energy I had left for what lay ahead.

Those hours before transplant were filled with questions. Would the day's events lead to my death? Would I survive, but be debilitated with crippling fatigue, exhaustion and infections? Or would Eric's microscopic cells actually eradicate my leukemia and become the seeds of a new and transformed life ahead? This was either going to be the first day of my new life or the beginning of the end of it.

When the nurses were done prepping me for the procedure, I showered, shaved and generally tried to spruce myself up. It was impossible.

"Whatever," I said out loud as I looked at the bags under my eyes and my drawn pale face. "There are some things that just can't be fixed." Then I strolled next door to see Wayde Gallant.

He was in a bad way. As usual, he was in bed watching television, but now he was wearing an oxygen mask and breathing heavily. He was hiccupping a lot, but between bouts he was still able to get out a few words. His parents were with him.

"Looks like they're going to transplant me again," he said haltingly, "but they're waiting for this pneumonia to clear."

Wayde never complained. Through his entire treatment, I had never heard him so much as whimper once.

"They're going to transplant you today?" he asked.

"Yeah," I said, "right in the next room, neighbor. Put a little prayer in for me."

"Will do," he promised, his words muffled under his mask.

"Thanks, buddy," I said. "You take great care, pal."

He forced a nod.

Before I left, I gave his parents a hug. I would have hugged Wayde too, but neither of us had any immunity left. We could have cross-infected each other. So I just sent him a reassuring glance. He nodded again, appreciatively, then turned his gaze back to his television. I knew he was elsewhere. He had come through so much already and there was still more to come. I quivered at the thought of going through another conditioning for a second transplant. Wayde was a stronger man than I.

Silently, I returned to my room. Just before noon, Patti Mayer floated in. She brought specially designed wrist magnets to ease my nausea and instructed Cecilia on the finer points of acupressure to help settle my stomach. With the right amount of pressure applied in the proper places, she explained, a little relief could be but a touch away. I did not have the heart to tell her I would likely need a few tons of pressure to get me through the next few weeks and that this was not going to be your average, garden-variety upset stomach. Actually, I was more concerned about the pain I had been told to expect when the mucous membranes throughout my body began to strip away because of the high dose chemotherapy. That, I had been told, could be extremely uncomfortable.

Weeks before, Cecilia had asked Rita if it might be possible for her to be my nurse that day. Rita had, after all, been there at the beginning. We thought it would be reassuring to have her there for another new beginning. She made special arrangements to make it happen.

When Rita arrived, we went for a short walk down the hall. I had spent a lot of time in bed the previous few days, had eaten almost nothing and was less than steady on my feet. But within a minute or so, I was amazed at the transformation. I actually felt pretty strong – relatively speaking.

"How are you feeling?" Rita asked in her usual sweet way.

"Well, aside from light-headed, I'm more apprehensive than anything else," I replied. "I know it's silly to worry about something completely outside my control, but sometimes, you know, I'm just not as good at it as I wish I was."

"That makes perfect sense," she affirmed, sliding her hand into mine. "I would be much more concerned if you said you were gung-ho."

"How could anyone be gung-ho after conditioning?" I asked.

"Someone who is in denial and trying to hide something," she said.

"What is there to deny?" I asked. "I'm undeniably weak and frightened. What's the sense in hiding it?"

"There isn't any," she agreed, "and that's a healthy state for you to be in right now."

She said nothing else. She just walked with me a while. I did so enjoy her ability to know when to be quiet and when to speak. It seemed to be one of her many talents. She had a wealth of knowledge and experience, but sometimes she just let it speak through silence.

When we got to the end of the corridor, she handed me a little note.

"Believe in yourself, Alan," it said. "Believe you are going the right way. We believe in you."

I gave her a big hug and thanked her for everything she had done. As usual, she brushed it off as nothing. We returned to our stroll.

"Rita," I finally said a minute or so later, "I have to ask you something."

"Yes? And what's that?"

"Well," I said, teetering on the brink, "it's about the two me's."

"Really? I've never met the other 'me.' Who's he?"

"He's the guy on the mountain," I explained. "You know, the adventurer guy."

"Yes," she hesitated as understanding began to creep into her voice. "I've heard about him, but you know, he's not here right now."

"Who exactly *is* here right now?" I asked.

"Well, you – a little tired, a little weak, but just you, no one else."

"And how do you know it's me?" I inquired.

She stopped, smiled and turned to face me.

"Alan," she said. "I know you for you. I know you to be a kind, sensitive and determined man. You are not what you do. You are who you are."

"That's good," I said, trembling a little. "Because I'm not sure if that other guy will ever come back after this."

"He might, he might not," she said candidly. "Or he might come back as a different guy, a stronger guy."

"That would be great," I prayed.

"Yes it would be, Alan," she concurred. "It definitely would."

I hoped she was right.

Just before 2 o'clock, Eric arrived. It was a joy to see him. He was robust and smiling and, as usual, joking.

"So," he said, turning to one of the nurses hanging over me as I lay in bed, "how soon can we expect this guy to become an over-stressed, round-faced businessman and start craving cigars, whiskey and cognac like me?"

"Well," Rita responded, "it'll take at least a couple of weeks."

"Good," Eric said. "I'll start to make plans right away then. I can put in an order for more Colts this afternoon and book a fishing trip for the end of the month. He should at least be able to bait a hook by then."

Everyone chuckled. It was classic Eric. Between quick one-liners and his insistence on repeatedly buffing my bald head, he was as he always was – absolutely loveable.

At exactly 2 p.m., "they" arrived. A lab technician pushing a vat of warm water on wheels walked into my room carrying three small plastic bags filled with what looked like frozen peach juice. They could have come straight out of the kitchen freezer down the hall.

"Look, Eric," I pointed out. "You've arrived again, but you're frozen solid."

"Not for long," the lab technician said, preparing to immerse one of the bags in the basin.

Each of the bags was about the size of a small Ziploc bag, but it seemed like they should be much bigger. They were so small compared to the power they held. "A new life is going to come out of those little things?" I wondered to myself. It was unbelievable.

Rita and the charge nurse, Kim, prepared me for the transplant. Carefully, they checked the serial numbers on the bags, cross-referenced them with the number on my hospital bracelet, took my pulse, blood pressure and temperature every few minutes, and handed me a roll of breath mints.

"What are these for?" I asked.

"Well," Rita explained, "you may actually get an unusual taste in your mouth during the infusion."

"You mean adult blood stem cells are like caviar?" I asked.

"Well, I guess that depends if you like caviar," Rita replied.

"I've never tasted it," I confessed.

"And our hope is you'll never have to taste these little guys again either," she countered.

"I'm with you there!" I replied emphatically.

Slowly, the lab technician, Judy Ranson, lowered the first bag of Eric's stem cells into the vat. As it had spent the last five weeks frozen at minus 180 degrees [C] in liquid nitrogen, it sent up mysterious vapors, like dry ice the moment it makes contact with air. Liquid nitrogen, I knew from my father's science experiments, actually boiled at room temperature.

"That's a funky effect," I said motioning towards the basin. "It looks like a cross between a magic show and a science experiment."

"That's an apt description," Rita agreed, never taking her eyes off what she was doing. "It's a bit of medical magic and the science of transplant. Actually, what Judy's doing is warming Eric's cells to your body temperature. That way you won't have ice flowing through your veins."

"I wouldn't want that," I said. "I had enough of that on Everest. Besides, it might make for a rude awakening if a chunk made its way to my heart. No ice blocks, please. We don't want any crash carts in here. I'm close enough as it is."

Judy handed the first bag to Kim, who called out its serial number and Eric's donor number as the bag went up on my I.V. pole. Once again, Rita carefully cross-checked the number with the one on my hospital bracelet. Meanwhile, Cecilia recorded the whole scene with a video camera so my parents could see and hear what happened. While Eric stood at my bedside, Bolek looked on from across the room. Patti sat quietly on a chair next to my bed. She never stopped smiling.

"Start chewing those mints," Rita reminded, putting her hand on my shoulder. "This will all be over before you know it."

I pulverized the mint in my mouth and waited for the taste of a transplant...

Nothing.

A hush fell over the room.

"How do you feel?" Rita asked about a minute later.

"Just fine," I said. "I can't taste Eric."

"If it tastes like alcohol, that's me," he jested.

We laughed again.

Within minutes, the contents of the first bag had disappeared into me.

With seasoned precision, Judy withdrew the second bag from the curling vapors and Rita and Kim put it up on the pole. Again the serial number and donor number were cross-checked. Again my pulse, blood pressure and temperature were taken. Rita and the other nurses watched me like hawks.

"Do people ever have a reaction to adult blood stem cells?" I asked, chewing diligently on my mints.

"Sometimes," Rita replied. "That's why we sedate you prior to the process. We prefer to be proactive rather than reactive."

"Good thing," I concurred. "It would be easier to chase Eric from the room rather than try to get rid of him once he's in my blood."

"He's in there for the moment," Rita said. "His genes are about to become a part of you."

Now *that* was something to contemplate – my brother's DNA inside me. I was okay with my mother's and father's, but my brother's as well? The concept was mind-boggling.

Someone else was now flowing through my veins for the first time. He was passing through my heart, running through my lungs, filtering through my organs – literally moving through every physical part of me. I wondered if cells had souls, because if they did, two souls were now merging together in what we hoped would be a birth, not of another human being, but of an entirely new blood and immune system starting from blood cell one. That, we prayed, would be a rebirth for me.

I thought I was a good soul and I knew Eric was. How could two good parts not make a successful healthy whole together? I guess that is where the paths of spirituality and science either grew closer together or drifted further apart – somewhere inside me at that moment.

I would like to tell you the transplant was this magnificent event, that it overflowed with excitement and euphoria like people imagine it does when you finally step to the summit of Everest after thirty-nine years of preparation. It was not. It was a mechanical act, just like taking those last steps to 29,035 feet had been. What made that day's final steps meaningful was exactly what had made those snowy steps meaningful too. It was not the steps themselves, but all the steps that had gone before – the months of discomfort, anxiety and fear during treatment, but more importantly, the Herculean efforts of the thousands of people who had made the day possible – everyone from the nurses and doctors to the administrators, lab technicians, psychologists, porters, geneticists and janitors. And, lest we forget, all those other climbers who had gone before me as well, those who had pushed science forward and those who had died in the process. Everyone had played a part. Just like reaching the top of the world, it had been a massive team effort. Someone had carried our tent, oxygen and food. They had washed my sheets. They had helped me bathe. We had climbed on their shoulders and now, thanks to them, we were standing on the threshold. We could not see the horizon from where we stood but we could see the humanity. It was all around us.

"I'm starting to feel a little flushed," I announced a few minutes after the second infusion.

"That's my red wine flush," Eric countered. "It's working already. How do we know when he's over the legal limit?"

"When it starts coming out his nose," one of the nurses retorted.

We roared.

The third bag came and went uneventfully and by 2:30 p.m., just thirty minutes after it had started, the transplant was over. It was completed so quickly we barely had a chance to appreciate what was happening. The nurses had done this so many times before it seemed like they could do it in their sleep. Of course they were completely alert, watching everything. For me, the transplant was just a few more bags on my I.V. pole – except they were *very* special bags.

"They can't take it out of you if it doesn't work, can they?" Eric asked.

"No," Rita said, "but it'll work."

"It *will* work," Eric echoed.

Somehow I expected to feel different, but it did not happen. What did happen was everyone sang "Happy Re-Birthday." It was fantastic, but a part of me wondered if I would live to see my first real "re-birthday." Just like I had on the summit of Everest, I now wondered if I could get down off the peak safely. If the up was over, that meant there was still the down.

Cecilia left the room to call my parents and let them know things had gone smoothly. I dozed intermittently, nodding off for a few minutes, then jerking suddenly awake, realizing something momentous had just happened, but knowing the climb was far from over.

At 5 p.m., Dale came by. He had been conspicuous in his absence during the transplant, but previous commitments had prevented him from being there. He had such timing. When he arrived, I was experiencing a mild case of rigors. Cecilia called for a nurse, did her cat-on-kitten pounce thing again and tried her best to comfort me. The nurse gave me Demerol and those glorious heated blankets, and in a few minutes the symptoms subsided.

"Christ, Hobson," Dale declared in his usual loving, sarcastic tone as he held me with Cecilia, "there you go again. No sooner am I in the door than we have to call for the nurse. I know I'm not the most handsome guy in the world, but you could try to be a bit more subtle."

Then he lowered his voice and whispered in my ear: "Congratulations, Al. I love you. I'm here for you."

Dale stayed with me until I had calmed down. We told him how well things had gone and that now it was just wait and see. He stayed about an hour, then bid us goodbye.

By 9 p.m., I was completely spent. Cecilia kissed me goodnight, gave me a very long, slow hug and told me how much she loved me. I felt it all the way to my heart. As a pigeon cooed outside my window and peered in at me lying listlessly in my bed, I slowly drifted off to sleep.

A whole new adventure had begun.

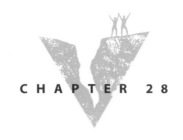

CHAPTER 28

Cecilia
VOTING FOR LIFE

A few days after the transplant, I enter Alan's hospital room, give him a kiss and take his breakfast out of my backpack and cooler. It has been several days since he has been able to eat and he is losing weight. The drugs he is receiving are stripping away the lining of his digestive tract, leaving his mouth and throat so painfully sore that he has been readmitted to Unit 57. The doctors have recommended he be put on morphine.

Today is Canada's federal election, and Alan is adamant about voting. I am confident there will be a voting station set up at the hospital for those patients who cannot go outdoors. I tell him I will get the details.

I hurry down the stairs and through the long hall connecting the Special Services Building to the main hospital. At the information window in the foyer, I stand in line behind worried faces. When I am face to face with the young girl in the booth, she smiles and asks calmly, "What can I do for you?" I smile back and say, "I'm looking for the voting booth so that my husband can vote." Her facial expression changes and I don't like the look she gives me. She says there is no voting booth in the hospital. I say, "Well how can patients vote today?" She says, "The voters' registrar office passed out absentee ballots last week. Your husband should have completed one then."

Instantly, I am furious. I snap back at her, "Well I guess we were out on a day pass when they came by. Are you telling me that that was my husband's only chance to vote?" She says that unless we go to our designated voting station, yes. This is not what I want to hear. I want to hear that the polling station is in the next hall or in the cafeteria. I want to hear there is a safe, protected place where Alan can vote.

I lower my head and turn away. I will have to tell Alan he can't vote today. When I arrive at his bedside, I whisper my findings into his ear and ask if he would like some crushed ice. He glares at me and says, "Then we have to go to the polling station." I fire back that I don't think that's advisable considering his condition.

He calls a nurse in and asks if he can go out. She says she'll have to check with the doctor and consult Alan's medication schedule, but she doesn't see why not. I am becoming more anxious every minute. Danger alarms are ringing in my head. Alan hasn't eaten in days, he is weak, he is on morphine and he doesn't have an immune system. How can he possibly go out to a crowded polling station?

The nurse comes back and offers us a two-hour pass. If Alan will wear a surgical mask to protect him from any airborne infections, he is free to go. When Alan makes up his mind to do something, he does it. With my heightened level of anxiety, all I can see are those WASH YOUR HANDS signs everywhere in the hospital. If we need to take such precautions here, how on earth are we going to protect him at a public polling station?

I relent and begin to pack the necessary things for our trip. He will need his wallet and driver's license, his voter registration card, coat, hat and our trusty blue basin.

Soon, we are ready to leave. The nurse hands us several surgical masks and gives Alan instructions. "Use one on the way to the polling station, one while at the polling station and one for the return," she says. With that, we proceed to the car.

Alan is a little lightheaded from the weight loss and morphine. As we are leaving the hospital, he reaches for a doorknob. I stop him with an abrupt "What are you doing?" He is startled. I say, "You don't have an immune system. You're not supposed to touch anything." He glowers at me and tells me to back off, that I'm being overzealous. "Overzealous!" I scream, "I'm only trying to save your life." I am walking close by his side when he pushes me aside to spit out some phlegm. I move away in anger and we both walk silently to the car.

Who is this man? Is it the morphine? Am I jeopardizing his life by driving him to the polling station? What is happening?

Eventually, Alan votes. We are still not talking on the way back to the hospital when all of a sudden he begins to gag. He lifts the basin to his face and gags again. This time, it sounds different. I am driving along a busy road when I realize he is unable to breathe. I quickly pull into a parking lot, jump out of the driver's seat and rush around to the passenger side. Alan is out of the car on all fours, his face down in the basin. The sound of the cars speeding by on the street only serves to quicken my heartbeat. My earlier anger is replaced by terror. As he continues to gag, a million thoughts flash through my mind simultaneously. Do I begin the Heimlich maneuver? He doesn't have any platelets, so if I dislodge his central line, he could bleed to death before I get him back to the hospital. Is he going to die right here in a parking lot? After what seems like an hour, but in reality is only seconds, the obstacle in his throat is ejected and the nightmare ends.

Snow begins to fall. It quiets the scene. The rush of blood flowing through my head eases. I dispose of the contents of the basin, walk back to the car where Alan is quietly sitting in the passenger seat and start the engine. We calmly return to the safety of the hospital.

The day's events have left both of us exhausted. I surrender Alan to the care of the nurses. He quickly falls asleep and I go home to relax. On the drive home, emotions overwhelm me, first anger, then hopelessness. Driving in a daze, I watch the flow of the Bow River and think about how close Alan came to drowning today, not in the icy waters of the river, but in his own bodily fluids. I realize I am ill-prepared to deal with such incidents. I vow to take an emergency preparedness course right away.

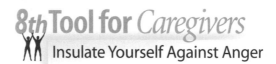

8th Tool for *Caregivers*
Insulate Yourself Against Anger

With the adrenalin out of my system, I stagger into the apartment, drop my backpack and cooler and head for the bedroom. I think about taking a nice soothing bubble bath but even that seems like too much effort. I'm emotionally spent. All I can do is flop on the bed.

While I'm lying there, the day spins before me. I realize Alan wasn't pushing me aside at the hospital. He was pushing aside cancer, the confinement and the loss of control. The day wasn't about voting at all. It was about taking back his life.

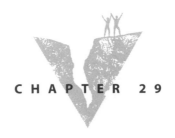

CHAPTER 29

Alan
INTO AND OUT OF THE CREVASSE

"You knew it was a matter of survival. You had to get there.
You didn't bother entertaining the consequences if you didn't.
All your energy now went into the next step."

– Sharon Wood,
First North American Woman to Climb Mt. Everest,
One Step Beyond

Incredibly, the day after my transplant I was able to go home on a day pass. There was no long isolation period during which I had to live in a plastic tent sequestered from the world of viruses, bacteria and fungi; no solitary confinement from even my closest friend's tender touch. Thanks to recent medical advances and the maverick style of Jim Russell and his team, at least one hurdle in the transplant challenge had been eliminated.

Both Cecilia and I were understandably tired. The minute we returned to the apartment, I went straight to bed. While I slept, Cecilia continued to work – doing the laundry, washing the dishes, cleaning the apartment, returning phone calls, paying bills, filling in disability insurance forms and making multiple copies of the video of my transplant to give to family and friends. When I awoke, she was ready as always to ply me with food. It is impossible for me to say exactly how much work she did because I slept through most of it at first. Her love was like a fountain. Once in a while, it would lose pressure and not rise to its maximum height, but most of the time it was a steady stream of strength.

Now began the anti-rejection drugs. Neoral, the drug used in most organ transplants, was used to suppress what little was left of my body's feeble immune system so Eric's incoming stem cells could establish a toehold. I consumed dozens of pills daily and did exactly what the doctors and nurses told me to do. Jim Russell stayed in the background, but he was undeniably present. The moment there was a hint of something untoward, he was on the telephone to us. If we were at the hospital, he was at my bedside in minutes. If we needed him, he was there. If we did not, he was busy tending to others who did.

The process of introducing foreign adult blood stem cells into a body is both science and art. I was given medications daily either to speed up or slow down the microscopic matchmaking. The method was very similar to the docking of a ship. Initially, there were special drugs that acted as forward engines to move my cells and Eric's closer together, then other drugs – "backwards engines" – that slowed things down. Bit by bit, day by day, our two entities made closer contact. I quickly realized that this docking process was well rehearsed. Jim and his transplant team followed a strict protocol, the result of decades of research and clinical trials.

Two days after my transplant, I visited Wayde Gallant. Thankfully, he seemed a little better and I was encouraged. We talked about his love of restoring old cars and made plans to take a spin in his latest restoration sometime in the spring when both of us had been discharged. He showed me a photo of his labor of love – a bright orange Dodge Challenger. Even from beneath his oxygen mask, his muffled voice communicated his passion for bodywork, paint and turning a wrench. I wondered if there was any way to get that passion into his hospital room, perhaps with a model or a radio-controlled car. He had a reason to live and I knew he would continue to eat even if it was difficult. Wayde would not fold. Like Rod, Wayde would drive his car until the gas tank was empty. You could see it in his eyes. They were dull and sunken, but they still reflected a dream of life. All he needed was an oil change and he would be back on the road.

The next few days came and went uneventfully. Cecilia and I would report to the hospital at 8 a.m., receive my medications and be gone by 1 p.m. after rounds. Then I would have a nap at home for a few hours, try to summon up the energy to go out for a walk or a very short bike ride, have a little to eat, watch some mindless television and collapse into bed for the night. The level of fatigue was extreme. I had a recurring fear that what the doctor had told us prior to transplant would actually come true – that I would be alive and breathing after transplant, but devoid of any energy with which to actually *live* life, and that things might never get better.

I had to do something. I had learned on Everest that if I got in the habit of lying around in my tent all day feeling dead, I could eventually end up that way. So in our apartment I set my mind to move beyond breathing. I focused everything I had on overcoming my own inertia. When I had had ten or twelve hours rest, I forced myself out of bed. I reprogrammed my mind to understand that after a certain point, fatigue was not always the result of insufficient sleep. Fatigue was the result of insufficient activity. I needed to re-oxygenate and re-energize my body, not lie around expecting that one day I would wake up and magically have all my energy back. That was not going to happen. It was an illusion, the same way the summit of Everest looked so close you could reach out and touch it from more than half a mile away. No, I needed to stop thinking I was tired and start acting like I could get stronger.

It was during this period that one of the recurring motifs of my earlier life came back to haunt me. To that point in my life, I had always been able to use my mind to make my body do what I wanted. Now that mindset began to work against me. No longer could I compare the performance of my present body with the one I had had in the past. It was like that house had been gutted by fire. Save for the bald head, I looked much the same on the outside, but inside I was radically different. Slowly, I emerged into a new understanding, one in which my only measure of success was not what I had been able to do last year, but what I had been able to do in the last hour. Even that, I soon discovered, sometimes did not always serve me. My energy level varied from minute to minute. Now my body, not my mind, dictated what I could do next.

This was completely uncharted territory for me. The concept of mind over matter, something deeply ingrained in my Type-A personality, was now completely ineffective for me. In fact, it was dangerous. Much as I might have wished to be able to will my body to do something, it was completely incapable of doing it.

It took all my mental fortitude to force myself to move, but even more to accept that whatever I could do at that moment was enough. For the first time in my life, good enough *had* to be good enough. Perfectionism, or what I would later come to know as "performance tyranny," was exactly that – tyrannical. If I decided my performance during an activity was inadequate, I might become my own worst tyrant. I had to be easier on myself. It had to be good enough just to be alive and to make my best effort. There was no past and no future. There was only the present. I either accepted that or I faced my most daunting adversary – myself.

The distance from the bed to the bathroom, roughly fifteen feet, felt like a mile. To go from there to the living room sofa was a marathon. I would find myself swaying down the hall steadying myself against the walls, my head swimming and my steps uncertain. I felt like I was at 27,000 feet.

Patience, it has been said, is a virtue, but it is one I do not possess. I felt physically hesitant and psychologically insecure. Emotionally, I was a wreck. My memories of hiking up and down mountains vanished into obscurity. *That* person seemed so distant from this one that it seemed impossible he could be the same man. And that was the point – he was not. Comparing myself with him set me up for failure. No, if I was going to climb this new mountain, I was going to have to redefine myself and build a new measuring stick for the new me, not one 29,000 feet high, but one twenty-nine feet long – the distance from my bed to the sofa.

I did not react well to this challenge. I became irritable and cantankerous. Within days, Cecilia and I were at odds with each other. When I roared, Cecilia withdrew. She took the brunt of the barrage because she was straight in the line of fire. It quickly became obvious we had to get outside. The question was how? If I was having a hard time getting across the apartment, how could I hope to get across the street?

I remembered Rod Barnes. He had done it by throwing back the sheets. So I took the first step – I got out of bed. Once this was accomplished, I somehow got dressed, and together Cecilia and I got ourselves to the elevator. Down we went, twenty-nine floors. I rested when we got to the ground floor. From there, we moved out to the car where I took another rest and from there, we drove to the Bow River west of downtown.

The minute I got out of the car, breathed in the fresh air and looked up at the trees, I felt a surge of energy. A short distance away was a trail. There amidst the swaying spruce, the pungent pine and the chirping of the squirrels, I once again reconnected with nature and as I always had, drew strength from her. I managed to get my body to move, rejoiced in the sweet smell of dry leaves intermixed with the snow and forgot for a minute that only an hour earlier, I had believed I could not get out of bed. It was a huge victory and it reaffirmed what I had heard – that people's health improves when they are surrounded by nature. It did not even have to be a forest. It helped if they could just look at a tree through an open window or contemplate the natural scene in a painting like the ones Debbie Baylin and her Art à la Carte team had supplied to us weeks earlier. That, and focusing only on the next step, were all that mattered.

The next day, the respite ended. What started as a sore throat quickly deteriorated into a feeling that my entire digestive tract was on fire. I could not swallow or even sip water. This was the start of mucositis, a condition in which the lining of the tract is slowly stripped away by the after-effects of high dose chemotherapy.

Quickly, I was readmitted to 57. After powerful oral painkillers failed to give me any measurable relief, we met with Jim.

"So, my friend," he observed, "you've got those horrid mouth sores? Awful stuff that. Unfortunately, it's to be expected. The conditioning has done its thing and all the bacteria from top to bottom are now going to have a little party at your expense. The bad news is it will probably last a few days and hurt like the dickens. The good news is a little morphine might really help."

Morphine? What the heck was he talking about? They gave morphine to car accident victims and drug addicts. This was just a really, really sore throat.

Jim read me instantly.

"No, Alan," he interjected before I even had a chance to say a word, "this is not about you acquiescing. This is about you convalescing. A little morphine might go a long way to helping you right now. You won't be taking it long enough to get addicted and we'll monitor your use of it very closely. It's your call, but many patients find it's invaluable through this stage of the transplant. It'll be okay."

What was there about this guy Russell? He would just peer at you over his glasses, smile softly and speak assuredly. He never told you what to do. He would just tell you the truth in such a way that you invariably accepted his advice.

The next five days were very uncomfortable. I did take the morphine and just as Jim had said, it did help. The nurses let me administer it using a little pump at my bedside. Studies have shown that patients who have control of their medication use less.

By the middle of the second night, however, I found myself hallucinating. Once on Everest, exhausted and unable to sleep properly due to the lack of oxygen at high altitude, I had awakened in the middle of the night in my tent swearing I saw balloon people decapitating each other with swords. Fortunately, through my drug-induced haze at the hospital, I somehow remembered this and recognized that my condition was starting to get out of control. I alerted the nurse. She disconnected me from the morphine and gave me a non-narcotic painkiller until my head cleared. Soon the demons disappeared and it was safe for me to go back on the morphine again.

The physical pain I was experiencing as a result of the mucositis was the least of my concerns. I knew that if I could not eat and I lost even five more pounds, my percentage of body fat would fall to near zero. I also knew from previous experience with weight loss that when I reached that level, I might begin to think and act irrationally. I tried not to envision what kind of a maniac I would become then, compounded with the one I already was on morphine.

Unfortunately, my worst fears came to pass. Dr. Hobson soon became Mr. Hyde. Sleep-deprived, unable to eat or drink, and on morphine, I gradually began to transform into something of a monster. When I learned from Cecilia that there was nowhere in the hospital where I might vote in Canada's federal election, I insisted on going to a public polling station. As I had no immune system, this was a foolish and potentially life-threatening decision, yet I refused to be dissuaded. Cecilia and I almost came to blows over it. While returning from casting my ballot, I nearly choked to death on a piece of dislodged throat lining. This episode, combined with the damage my toxic and mercurial personality did to our relationship, produced icy relations between Cecilia and me for several days afterwards. During this period, the mucositis worsened to the point where I became unable to speak. So I communicated silently using a note pad. For everyone around me, it was probably just as well.

Still, it was lonely. I came to understand what it must have been like for my nephew, Michael, to have been confined to an isolated room for weeks after his bone marrow transplant. I meditated as much as I could, although I found that concentrating was difficult in my swimming psychological state and even sitting up to focus on anything was extremely uncomfortable. My digestive tract just did not want to bend. So I lay there almost immobile, staring at a point on the ceiling, drifting in and out of sleep. Cecilia and I did anything but flow. We tried to hang on, if not to each other, then to hope that we could crawl out of this emotional pit.

A few days later, although I still could not eat or drink, my voice gradually returned. That was marvelous. I chatted freely with the nurses and for the first time in days could tell Cecilia that I loved her in my own words. I was also able to apologize to her for my outbursts of anger and frustration during the voting debacle. Helen MacRae had warned us that whatever happened while the survivor was on narcotics had to be forgotten, but it would be hard to forget my callous irrationality on voting day. I would regret it for a long time, and it was weeks before I was able to forgive myself. Fortunately, it did not seem to take Cecilia that long. She saw me for what I was – a tired, frightened, frustrated, drugged-up, underfed and confined survivor who wanted his life back, but who was not likely going to get his way for some time, if ever.

In fairness, my anger was not all drug-induced. There was still a lot of pent-up hostility toward cancer and the immobility and loss of control it had created in my life. The disease produced a shocking role reversal: a strong-willed, independent person like me suddenly became dependent. In addition, the unrelenting uncertainty and fatigue had made Cecilia susceptible to caregiver burnout. There is a direct link between cancer and marital breakup and it is easy to see why. By changing those it touches, it changes how they touch each other.

The next day, the physical tide turned. My blood tests showed an increase in the number of platelets, the first indicator that engraftment might have started. Now, almost two weeks after transplant, I found I could swallow again and over the next few days, thanks to an increase in my white blood cell count, there was a gradual improvement in my oral health. Soon I could eat solid food, although because of the drug conditioning, I still could not taste it.

Two days later, the miracle happened. All my blood cell counts rocketed up. With every passing day, they rose higher and higher, and with them, my spirits. On day fifteen, we learned I would be discharged the next day to Unit 57B, the one for day patients. We felt positively liberated. We knew the engraftment could still fail, or acute Graft Versus Host Disease could set in, or a relapse could occur, or, or, or…but we lived in the moment.

We were alive and rebuilding and thankful. Even a heavy head cold could not stop Cecilia from sharing the joy with me. From beneath a hospital mask, she continued the outpouring of love and commitment that had become her hallmark. Her anxiety level dropped, and for the first time in weeks, she relaxed a little. As a couple, we returned to a state of partial stability.

Jim came by and confirmed the news.

"Engraftment has begun," he said with guarded optimism. "It's looking really good, right on schedule. Time for you two to get out of here for a while."

I called Eric to give him the news. As usual, I was not able to actually speak with him since he was immersed in an endless stream of intense business meetings, so I left him a message.

"Just wanted to let you know, Brother, that your stem cells have found a home in me and they're starting to make babies," I said. "I didn't know you could bear children, Eric, but I think you should tell Bunny [his wife Diane's nickname] in case she'd like to let you take over as the family matriarch for a while."

Then I called my parents.

"One of your sons appears to be in the preliminary stages of saving your other son's life. If there was ever a time when there was strength in numbers, this appears to be it."

"Yippee!" my mother squealed like a school girl let out for recess. "That's great! That's just great!"

"Well done, Son!" Dad hollered in an unusual display of emotion. "We're pulling for you, kid."

By noon, Cecilia and I were on our way home. After lunch, I lay down for my usual nap. Cecilia snuggled in next to me on the bed and we held each other close. Whatever the future held, we did not care. We were home and we were together. Blood cell counts vanished into insignificance. The only thing that counted was the joy of life and the life that we still had – bent but not broken, weakened but still strong.

A stillness fell over downtown as the late afternoon turned to evening.

Then, far off to the west, on the other side of the apartment window, came the eventual glow of sunset. Somewhere beyond the horizon, we hoped, there was our journey's end.

I put my nose up against the pane and pushed it toward the twilight. Suddenly, the quarter-inch mile seemed shorter. The cold glass gave a bit.

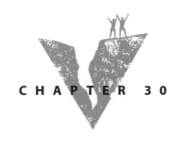

C H A P T E R   3 0

Cecilia
THE UPHILL
GRIND

I am the type of person who needs to define the goal, make my list of things to do, check the items off as they're done and move to the next goal. Our time in the hospital had several goals. We met each one and moved to the next. The first goal was to put the leukemia into remission after the first round of chemotherapy. The second was to go through treatment with as few infections as possible. The third was to successfully endure the adult blood stem cell transplant. This we did with flying colors.

With so many triumphant accomplishments, I am overjoyed when Alan is discharged.

We quickly gather up all our belongings. Two trips to the car and we're ready to go. Even though we are carrying heavy loads from Alan's room, we bounce down the hall to the elevators. We drive home with the windows down. A light snow is falling and I try to catch a snowflake on my tongue at the stoplight. I'm sure the driver next to me thinks I'm crazy, but I don't care. I'm enjoying the crisp cold air and the fresh taste of freedom.

I open the door to the apartment thinking how fabulous it is to be home for Christmas. Now, we will get back to a "normal" life – no running to and from the hospital, no more living on hospital time. We are home. We'll be sleeping together in our own bed. Our life together will continue. We'll *have* a life together.

The days go by slowly. Without the schedule of the hospital, time seems to drift aimlessly. The goal becomes less immediate. Our goal is to live a year, then two, then five. Five is the benchmark for being successfully "cured."

We argue more frequently now. Alan still has to take several medications during the critical one hundred days post-transplant. He is virtually without an immune system and any infection could prove fatal. In addition, there is a fine balance to be achieved: the new adult blood stem cells must be allowed to take up residency in Alan's body but not to overwhelm his system. Hence the medications. One in particular, Neoral, an anti-rejection drug, is the most critical. As the discharge nurse told me, it must be taken around-the-clock on a strict schedule. I have my list of all the medications and the times they need to be taken.

It's Sunday afternoon and it looks like it might snow. We both need some laughter and watching a comedy sounds like the perfect way to spend the evening. Since Alan is not yet able to be among large groups in a confined area, we can't go to the theater. I tell him I will run down to the local video store to pick up something that will have us rolling on the floor. I grab my wallet and gently remind Alan to take his medications in five minutes. He says, "Okay."

Our office is right down the street from the video store, so I decide to stop in, check emails and get a little work done before I head back to the apartment. After spending a little less than an hour at the office, I head to the store. Once there, I find myself searching through dozens of comedies for a really good slapstick movie. Finally, I pick out several Monty Python classics and with laughter in hand, I walk back home.

I open the apartment door to find Alan sleeping on the sofa. I quietly tip-toe past him to the kitchen, where I find the Neoral and his other medications sitting on the kitchen table. A rush of anxiety passes through me. I quickly pour a glass of water and gather up the multicolored pills. I set the glass of water on the coffee table, kneel down and gently nudge him. "Alan," I say, "you have to wake up." He opens his eyes and glares at me. "You didn't take your medications at 5 p.m. It's now after 6." With anger in his voice, Alan snaps, "Stop treating me like a child. I'll take my medications when I'm ready." He turns away.

I try to explain that I feel a responsibility to his nurses, doctors, family and friends to ensure he makes it to the next goal. After all, they released him to my care. I will not let them down. I will not let *him* down. This is a critical time. Any infection could cost him his life.

Alan doesn't want to hear a rational explanation of why I awakened him to take his medications. He doesn't want to hear he has to take medications at all. For me, this is simply a necessity. For him, it's evidence he's still not in control.

The evening turns from what we hoped would be a marathon of laughter to a marathon of silence. Our normal life is slipping further away. The apartment soon becomes an extension of the hospital. I feel Alan withdrawing from me but I'm paralyzed. I've hit the wall and I don't know what to do. My past experience with cancer did not prepare me for the aftermath of treatment.

Alan no longer sees me as his partner in life. He views me as a nurse rather than a lover. How do I maintain my roles as friend, partner and lover when I am administering medications, cleaning his central line and holding a basin under his mouth as he loses the lunch I just prepared for him?

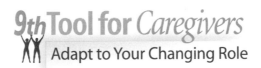

9th Tool for *Caregivers*
Adapt to Your Changing Role

We know we cannot continue like this. We again seek the help of Dr. Helen MacRae. During one of our sessions, Helen asks Alan if he has read *Dancing in Limbo – Making Sense of Life after Cancer* by Glenna Halvorson-Boyd and Lisa K. Hunter. He says no. Desperate for any information, I purchase the book at a local bookstore that afternoon and begin reading it that night. In the first chapter, I gain insight into what I didn't know and what Alan couldn't express. While I am focused on getting back to a life before cancer, Alan is disoriented and confused, "lost in the most familiar places," the book says.

I also turn to another book, *It's Not About the Bike*, by cancer survivor and then two-time Tour de France winner, Lance Armstrong, with Sally Jenkins, to try to get a better understanding of how other high achievers handle critical illness. It enlightens me as to what Alan the athlete might be feeling. One passage I find most revealing: *One definition of 'human' is as follows: 'characteristic of people as opposed to animals or machines, especially susceptible to weakness, and therefore showing the qualities of man.' Athletes don't tend to think of themselves in these terms; they're too busy cultivating the aura of invincibility to admit to being fearful, weak, defenseless, vulnerable, or fallible, and for that reason neither are they especially kind, considerate, merciful, benign, lenient, or forgiving, to themselves or anyone around them.*

I begin to understand how I am feeding this feeling of weakness. I have so much to learn.

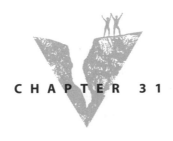

CHAPTER 31

Alan
STARTING TO
CRAWL

"Outstanding!" Dr. Chris Brown said as he glanced at my blood cell counts a few days after engraftment had begun. "You're right on track."

Cecilia and I were thrilled. We delighted in the moment, drinking it in like fine wine. In addition to being one of the team of a dozen or so oncologists who attended to me, Chris was also one of the nation's leaders in leukemia research. We would learn later that he was an avid cyclist and a vigorous proponent of physical activity in cancer prevention and recovery. We made it our goal to continue to give him reason for optimism.

The next stage of our expedition now began – the first hundred days post-transplant. If we could get through this period, we would not be out of the woods, but the chances of life-threatening complications would be lessened. It was now early December. If we could make it to February 23, we would have made a significant step in the right direction. That became out next goal.

Realizing the transplant process was taking a continuing toll on our relationship, Cecilia and I headed in to see Helen MacRae. By now, we were coming to know her well. Of Scottish descent, but without a brogue, she had piercing blue eyes, silver hair and a commanding personality. She spoke clearly and emphatically, and we valued her keen intellect and candor. Like

Dr. Poon, she had the guts to be direct, even if it hurt, and she did not hesitate to confront us on an issue if she believed we were not facing up to it. When it came to cancer, she seemed to believe that there was no point in beating around the bush. This time, with a few pointed and probing questions, she once again skillfully exposed some of the matters now troubling us.

"The other day a guy on the street saw us walking together," I recounted. "He saw Cecilia carrying a backpack full of food, medicine and clothes, and me carrying only my plastic barf basin. He said, 'What are you doing, man? She's carrying everything for you. What kind of a man are you?' For a moment my male ego was bruised, but it occurred to me he was right. Cecilia *is* carrying everything. All I seem to be doing is treading water. I abhor being treated like a child and worse still, I despise the feeling of going nowhere. I want to do things on my own, but at the moment all I seem to be able to do is subsist."

Cecilia responded with her usual clarity: "When you were on Everest," she asked, "did you let the Sherpas carry loads for you? Did they wash dishes, cook meals, fetch water and prepare the route? Of course they did. You didn't feel guilty then because you knew your role would come later on summit day. Well, this mountain is no different. While you're focused on getting better, I can be a Sherpa and take care of whatever I can. I'm just finding it challenging carrying the load, the same way you're finding it challenging sharing it."

Seeing her opening, Helen leaned forward. With her usual penetrating stare, she gave it to me straight from the hip: "Listen carefully to the messages you're giving yourself, Alan," she counseled. "You're saying 'I'm weak. I can't carry my load.' How about 'Thank goodness there is someone in my life who can carry the load for me now'? Do you know how fortunate you are Alan? Do you have any idea? I've seen lots of people sit in the same chair you're sitting in right now who climbed this mountain alone. Believe me, that is a much harder mountain to climb. If you think Everest was tough, try that one."

She was absolutely right. They both were. There was no denying that. But I still wrestled with my vulnerability. I was sick, or at least I felt sick. So I was forced to surrender. I did not like it, but I did it.

Convalescence was compromising ground. To reach what I had regarded as a physical goal – getting to the other side of the crevasse or to February 23 – I would now have to dig deeper inside myself to find a different strength. The situation reminded me of the words I had once heard from Sharon Wood, the first North American woman to climb Everest, when she had told me that to climb up, you actually had to reach down.

"I discovered it wasn't a matter of physical strength," she had told me during interviews for *One Step Beyond*, "but a matter of psychological strength. The contest lay within my own mind to penetrate those barriers of self-imposed limitations and get through to the good stuff – the stuff called potential, ninety percent of which we rarely use."

I too would now have to make that journey – not upwards, but inwards.

That weekend, Cecilia and I drove to the mountains. We found a room and collapsed into bed beside a fading fire. We slept soundly.

Saturday dawned to overcast skies and cool temperatures. We did not have a plan. The last four months had been so regimented by hospital cycles that it was great just to sleep in, roll out of bed and make it up as we went along. I was weak, but as always the power of the mountains rekindled my energy and ambition. Cecilia and I decided to try a hike up nearby Sulphur Mountain and see if either of us still had any legs left.

The moment we started up the trail and my respiration rate increased, I began to feel revived. Although far from feeling strong, I prized every breath of mountain air. I drew it into my body like food from the forest. I smelled the sweet scent of the trees, heard the shriek of the ravens circling overhead and delighted in the sight of fresh deer tracks at my feet. Our boots squeaked in the snow and within minutes, I was transformed from survivor to hiker, from infant to adult.

The steps came slowly and gingerly. What they lacked in strength, I made up for in memory. After months of confinement at home or in the hospital, I knew I had only to put one wavering foot in front of the other – and that was all.

The trail climbed gently to the top. When Cecilia and I popped out at the summit a little over ninety minutes later, we were surprised and delighted. Not wishing to push the envelope any further, we took the gondola down, gaped in awe at the view and enjoyed a simple celebratory bite at a local restaurant. The next day, after a short sightseeing trip to a nearby lake, we drove back to Calgary. On the way home, we allowed ourselves to fantasize about the future for the first time since my diagnosis. If there was one thing cancer had taken from us, it was the luxury to dream.

But a future together was so far ahead of us we could not dream for long. We were still climbing back from cancer, and for that we were grateful. We knew that there were many others who had never been given that gift. Still, there had to be a balance somewhere between gratitude and desire. Without desire, there was little reason to want to live, but without gratitude, there was no grace in that living.

On Monday morning, we reported to 57B for the usual drill – blood tests, vitals, a once-over of the body to check for signs of GVHD and instructions on how to take the next wave of medications. It was then that a nurse pulled me aside as I sat in one of the treatment rooms.

"I have some sad news, Alan," she said quietly. "I'm sorry to have to tell you that Wayde died early this morning of a hemorrhage."

I stared at the floor. For a long while, I just sat there, stunned.

"If it's any consolation, he didn't suffer," she continued. "His platelet count was very, very low and Dr. Russell had alerted his family to prepare for the worst. I'm so sorry, Alan. I know he was a friend."

I went numb. I just shook my head and said, "But we were going to go cruising in the spring. We were going to hop in his Challenger and charge down the highway. It was going to be such fun. It was going to be…"

My thoughts wandered off with my voice.

My mind went to the weekend Cecilia and I had just shared. I thought about what we had experienced. While we had been out blissfully sucking in the fresh mountain air and snacking on trail mix, Wayde had been taking his last breaths.

Why was I alive? Why had my transplant taken and Wayde's had not? Why had I had all the luck and all Wayde got was pneumonia? It did not make sense.

My mind spun on the injustice. I felt terrible guilt. Wayde was a great guy. He was unassuming and humble and kind. The world needed more people like him. Why had he been taken from us? Why was I still here?

Suddenly, reality was back – like a cold north wind when you break through the tree line. It blasted into my brain.

Cecilia did not know how to comfort me. How could she? She had deliberately not let herself become attached to the other patients the way I had. She had had enough foresight to know that sooner or later, something like this would happen. When it did, she knew at least one of us would have to be strong.

Stiffly, I stood and walked from the room. Cecilia just let me go. I headed for Jim Cleghorn's room and I sat down at the end of his bed. As usual, he was creating something, this time a logo for the new audio business he dreamed of starting if he got out of the hospital. We chatted for a while about his creation, then I told him about Wayde.

"They told me already," he said, his eyes downcast. "That sucks. That really sucks. It could have been you or me, Al."

That truth hurt as much as Wayde's death. Now, of the guys who had been admitted around the same time, there were only Rod, Jim, Andrew and me left. Wayde and my old roommate were gone. The statistics were cold and undeniable – one in three of us gone in less than six months. That was stark reality.

"What are you going to do now?" Jim asked.

"I don't know," I confessed. "I guess I'm just going to keep on until I can't keep on any longer. This whole experience frustrates the hell out of me. There's so much outside our control. It makes you wonder if anything's in our control."

"Sometimes not even our bladders," Jim replied. "You pee the bed and you wonder what the hell's going on. So, Al, what the hell's going on?"

"Damned if I know. All I can see is that some of us are living and some of us are dying and I have no idea why, but I'm told there's Someone who knows. The docs can tell us medically, but I sure can't tell you logically. Mostly, as far as I can see, we're all just trying to make it through the day."

Jim nodded.

"That's all anyone's doing," he affirmed.

"I guess you're right," I echoed.

I did not get it. I did not get it at all. It was not enough just to make it through the day. There had to be a purpose beyond that, some larger meaning. What was life without dreams, without goals and without some means of achieving them? Buddhists believe there is pure peace. If that is so, then death must also be peaceful – not the event, but the result, because death is the absence of desire. I prayed that was where Wayde was – basking serenely in the spring sunshine on the hood of his bright orange Challenger. Maybe he had realized he could go there without waiting. Maybe he had actually fulfilled his desire.

If there was one lesson I was supposed to be learning from this experience, it was that perspective was a key to truth. What I had taken for granted before cancer, I would never take for granted again. Cancer-related deaths, especially amongst fellow patients, would now become a regular part of our lives. With every announcement, we would again be reminded of our own fragile mortality.

Wayde was dead. I hated saying that. I hated saying it because I could just as easily have said "Alan is dead." But somehow I was alive. The confusion and the injustice mixed together bitterly.

Glumly, I returned to 57B.

Cecilia was just as I had left her – still sitting there, patiently waiting.

"What do we do now?" I mourned. "Wayde's gone."

"That's right, Alan," she said supportively. "Wayde is gone. That's sad.

It's very sad. He was a great guy, a decent guy, a kind guy. But we both learned something from him. We learned that the road can take a sudden turn at any time so it's best to hold on to what we have now. And all we have now is the only thing we've ever had – this moment. So as sad as this moment is, we can still remember that it is precious. At least we are alive to feel it."

After a few moments of silence, Cecilia finally added, "Wayde would be very disappointed if he thought we'd missed a moment. All we can do now is see if we can create some new moments. The problem is, now that you've expended your energy for the week and maybe the month after our hike, there isn't a lot left you can do three weeks out of transplant."

We did manage to create a new moment two days later. While I napped in the passenger seat, Cecilia drove to a woodlot in the foothills. There we found ourselves a delightful little Christmas tree. We laughed and joked that the tree was older than I was. Like me, it looked a little worse for wear, but we did not care. We put five dollars into the kitty as instructed, gave thanks that we lived in a place where you could still cut down your own tree, and stuffed the spruce into the back of our car.

That Christmas tree expedition would be another one of those precious moments we would hang on to when things got bad. Months before, neither one of us had been sure if I would even live to see Christmas. Although it was still three weeks away, we were hopeful we could make it.

On the way back to town, we stopped for homemade ice cream at a little shop in the town of Cochrane.

"One tall red raspberry shake to go, please!" I announced to the clerk.

"And would you like chocolate sprinkles on that?" she asked.

"Absolutely," I replied. "And whipped cream and M&M's and Maraschino cherries and Reese's Pieces and anything else you can throw in there."

"My, you're feeling pretty bold today," she observed, laughing.

"Not every day these days," I announced. "Not every hour or every minute, but at this moment, yes, I am. It's my bold new life plan: guilt-free living."

As I sipped on my shake on a bench with Cecilia, I relished the cool sensation on my dry coarse throat and thanked Baba for small mercies. I still could not taste a thing, but it did not matter. I was still tasting life as much as I could and as far as I could tell, that is what I was supposed to be doing.

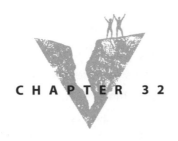

C H A P T E R   3 2

Cecilia
R E T U R N I N G   T O
" N O R M A L "

It is the first weekend in December and Alan suggests I go to a nearby spa for a relaxing massage as an early Christmas present. As wonderful as my massage had been at the couples' retreat, however, I feel like the apartment walls are closing in on me and the last thing I want is to be confined to a small room, even if it is for a massage. In any case, I've been so anxious lately that I don't feel like I could lie on the massage table and relax. I need to get outdoors and move. I suggest we drive to Banff for a short hike up Sulphur Mountain and a ride down on the gondola. A day in the mountains is just what we need. Alan agrees.

There are heavy clouds in the sky and I wonder if it will snow. I would welcome a good snowfall. I need to feel the snow on my face and hear it crunch beneath my feet. Just as a fresh snow covers the dirty streets with a shimmering white blanket of newness, I want the snow to cover the hurt and pain of the previous months.

The drive evokes memories of my visit to the Canadian Rockies two years earlier. I was awed at seeing the mountains for the first time. Everything was so new and we had such energy then. I want our relationship to be like those mountains around us – built on a solid base and reaching into a vast sky of possibilities.

We have a lovely time on the hike and stop for dinner at our favorite restaurant. I like the sense of normalcy the day brings. I don't feel like we are survivor and caregiver. I feel like we are a couple on a date.

I so desperately want things to be normal again. I want to put everything behind us and start fresh. With the transplant completed, we have successfully crossed the first hurdle. For the first time in six months, I am able to structure my day. I begin to go into the office on a more regular schedule. I start back exercising and I begin to make plans for next week. For me, this is comforting. I feel I can now look to the future, if only a little. So, I set my sights on Christmas.

December has always held a special place in my heart. It is a month filled with laughter, good food, time with friends and family and the joy of giving. I want our time to be what it was our first Christmas together – clean, fresh and full of wonder. It's only the first week in December, but I don't care. I want a Christmas tree. Not just any Christmas tree will do. This one has to be special. This tree will stand for happier times, hope for the future and gratitude for what we have.

I insist we go out and cut down our own tree. Alan turns to me with a curious look, then grins understandingly. He can see I'm serious.

I begin making phone calls to find out where we can go to cut down a tree. Alan begins to pack the necessary gear: a saw, rope to tie the tree onto the vehicle and, of course, the proper clothing to keep us warm while out on the hunt.

After a long drive, we bounce out of the car (well, actually, I bounce. Alan tries to.) With saw in hand, we take to the woods in search of the perfect tree. We are in a wilderness area the government of Alberta has designated for thinning. Only a certain size and type of tree may be cut to permit others around them to grow taller.

Carefully, we search the area for that special tree. We walk around in the snow looking at dozens of trees from different angles when Alan suddenly proclaims:

"Here, my love, I've found our tree."

Alan is standing next to a six-foot tall tree with small pinecones clinging to its branches. It doesn't look like the perfectly shaped specimens you see on the tree lots, and that's what I like best about it. It hasn't been groomed all year to perfection. It has been shaped by nature and it's real. This is vitally important to me. All through my childhood, we erected an artificial tree each Christmas. Each branch was perfectly crafted to look like the real thing. I hated having an artificial tree. It looked pretty, but there was no scent of pine in the air. And it had no life. I vowed then never to have a synthetic tree in my house. I wanted the real thing.

"It's perfect," I squeal with delight.

Alan kneels in the snow and begins exposing the trunk. Then he takes our little hand saw and slowly starts cutting. The trunk doesn't look very thick, but it takes each of us several turns to cut the tree down. Once it's felled, Alan takes hold of the bottom and I take hold of the top and we raise the tree to our shoulders. With the precision of a marching band, we walk proudly back to the car carrying our new symbol of happiness.

I have a vacuum flask of hot chocolate ready in the car. I pour out the sweet steaming liquid, and together we raise our plastic cups in a toast to hopes and dreams.

C H A P T E R   3 3

Alan
S T A N D I N G

"If you looked at the whole picture at once and what was involved it would completely exhaust you. But when you take it one step at a time, when you take one increment and work away at it, you can achieve great things."

– Mike Beedell,
Adventurer,
One Step Beyond

Our hike, combined with our little Christmas tree expedition, laid me flat for the rest of the week. I quickly learned that for every significant expenditure of energy, there was a greater price paid later in fatigue. It was as if I had no reserves on which to draw. With a blood system being rebuilt, I was asking a child to do a man's work. It would take time for that child to get stronger.

"You're like a baby whose parents opened a checking account the day you were born and put ten dollars into it," Helen MacRae explained in her usual wise way. "You don't have a savings account because you haven't been alive long enough to have accumulated any savings. All you have is what's in your checking account. Once the money in there is spent, it will take a while for it to come back. Your newest currency isn't cash, it's energy. You will need to learn to spend it wisely. A transplant creates a completely new energy awareness."

I recalled how on Everest I would often lie exhausted in my tent in base camp for hours trying to decide if I absolutely *had* to go to the toilet yet. I knew that to get out of my tent, stagger across the rocks and boulders to the windswept loo and stagger back would take a lot of effort. And because there was less oxygen pressure at that altitude, once my energy was expended, it would not come back until I returned to sea level. So I waited until the situation was almost desperate before I made the "dash" (no one dashes anywhere at high altitude).

"This is really hard," I wrote in my diary just a few days before Christmas. "I find myself having to stop all the time and lie down and sleep. A very simple task can take several days to complete and that is very frustrating…All the way around, this is a challenge."

It took almost as much mental energy to keep my mind from falling into the depression along with my body. I could decide to feel angry, sorry for myself, or just plain frustrated, or I could focus my energy on getting better. To get better, I concluded, I had to circulate oxygen to my muscles. With more oxygen would come more energy, I hoped, and with more energy would come more life. I had to move. I had to. If I did not, I would become imprisoned in our apartment just as I had to some degree been temporarily incarcerated in my hospital room.

So each day I willed myself to move – one more sheet thrown back, one more pair of pants donned, one more trip to the toilet completed. It was an inner Everest. The trip down the hall from the bedroom to the living room became a ridge and although it did not make my palms sweat with fear the way an exposed, windblown one did, it definitely raised my heart rate. A can of soup successfully heated was a slope ascended, staying standing in the shower long enough to wash my hair and dry off was an obstacle overcome, and a ringing telephone answered in time was a summit achieved. They were seemingly insignificant and simple steps, but they were the beginnings. They were, quite literally, baby steps. They were like the ones I had watched the Sherpas take on Everest – day after day, week after week.

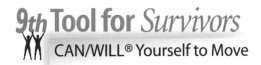

9th Tool for *Survivors*
CAN/WILL® Yourself to Move

"Slowly, slowly. No hurry," they would say. Eventually, this apparently simple strategy had worked. If the weather permitted, they had usually stood on top.

My friends, by and large, were completely unaware of our tedious struggle. They assumed, as I had, that once treatment was over, the crisis was over. Many of them stopped calling, and I found it difficult to summon up enough energy to call them. A few visited us from time to time, but mostly Cecilia and I marked time. We began to feel like we were stuck in a back eddy and the rest of the world was flowing right past us in the stream. Now we understood the phrase "mainstream society." We were out of it.

To redeem myself, when I had regained enough energy we would head out to the hills again. There I would haul myself to the top of a small peak. Then for days afterwards, I would ride the couch on the bottom of the energy cycle again. To some this might have seemed like a man beating his head against a wall. Actually, it was a man climbing a wall.

Everest had been a good teacher, but cancer was proving to be a better one. On Everest we would have to wait patiently for our bodies to acclimatize and for the weather to cooperate before making our summit bid. Now I would have to wait for my body to grow stronger and for my new blood to learn to carry more oxygen. The difference between the two mountains was the degree of patience required – on Everest it was a few weeks, but on my inner Everest it would be years.

Even though so far I was a survivor, my time on the couch taught me the patience of a patient. I learned that the challenge was mental as well as physical, and that unless I first learned how to slow down my mind and win the mental game, I would never be ready to speed up my body and win the physical one. For the endless hours I spent on the couch, I was no longer a human doing. I learned how to be a human being.

> *"I was no longer a human doing. I learned how to be a human being."*
>
> – Alan Hobson

While I certainly learned to be more patient with my body during my recovery, I never really mastered the art psychologically. As soon as my body showed any sign of strengthening, mentally, I drove it forward. It was not performance tyranny. It was CAN/WILL.

As I recovered on the couch between activity sessions, there were some fears I did not succeed in silencing. There were still bills to pay and an office to maintain, and I knew that without doing something to bring in income, we were eating into precious savings every day. We had decided to keep an office and skeleton staff going so that if I lived, we would have something to come back to. But if Cecilia and I survived this, would we be able to survive bankruptcy?

My friend, Dale Ens, who doubles as my financial advisor, caught wind of this and set me straight in an instant. He glared at me and said, "You're not losing money, you're buying your life back. The money you're spending now is being spent to buy back your future. You can thank your lucky stars you've got disability insurance coverage and enough in savings to see you through this for the time being, not to mention that wonderful woman of yours without whom you'd have probably stood a fool's chance in Vegas to have lived a day beyond your diagnosis. I love you to pieces, buddy, but for heaven's sake, keep your eye on the ball. The ball, in case you've missed it, looks a damned sight brighter today than it did four months ago, so quit dwelling on dollars and get on with the only business that's worth a cent to you or to anyone else right now – the business of healing."

A few days later, Jim Russell also told me something I needed to hear.

Unfortunately, I did not want to hear it. He diagnosed me with a mild case of Graft Versus Host Disease (GVHD). It presented itself as a slightly itchy rash over half my body.

"That's the bad news," he countered, trying to put a positive spin on the situation. "The good news is that it's just the right amount of Graft Versus Host Disease. We want just enough so that it's clear that your brother's new stem cells are manufacturing T-cells that are attacking any cancerous blasts left over after the chemotherapy.

"There's just one catch. To treat the Graft Versus Host Disease, we're going to have to put you on prednisone, a powerful steroid that has some rather unpleasant side effects."

"Like what?" I inquired.

"Well, if we have to keep you on it for too long, you could suffer serious bone degeneration. If that happens in the hip area, you might not be able to walk. On the other hand, the drug should increase your energy level. It'll definitely boost your appetite, which may cause you to put on weight, keep you awake at night with insomnia and produce rapid mood swings that could turn you into a bit of a bear."

"Even more than he already is?" Cecilia teased.

"Well, actually," Jim replied, "worse."

We discussed the alternatives, but there really were not many. If we did not do something, the GVHD might escalate into something more serious. Some weightlifters used steroids, I knew. When they bulked up, they also sometimes experienced "roid rage" – drug-induced explosive outbursts.

This was not that kind of steroid, Jim explained. It did not build muscle mass.

"But you said it could turn me into a bit of a bear," I persisted.

"That's right, Alan, it could," he admitted. "But you needn't be that way for long."

"For the sake of our relationship, I hope not," Cecilia observed.

Much as I hated to take yet another drug, we went home with a prescription. That afternoon, even before starting on prednisone, I felt angry.

First chemotherapy, then anti-fungals, antibiotics, anti-virals, anti-coagulants, anti-nauseants, anti-convulsants, anti-rejections, blood transfusions, rabbit hormones, cell growth stimulants, sleeping pills, morphine and now steroids. I had had it. I was maxed out on meds.

Sensing the need to release pent-up hostility from this further loss of control, I made an appointment to see Patti Mayer for some acupuncture. Instead of sticking me with needles, she performed an unusual procedure called "cupping." First, using a match, she lit a gauze pad soaked in alcohol and held the flaming wad for a second or two under an inverted transparent glass cup. Then she carefully placed the cup over a pre-selected point on my back. Thanks to the suction the technique created, the cup adhered tightly to my skin. With a half dozen or so other such tumblers, she repeated the process, placing each one in a different spot on my back. To my astonishment, within minutes, the skin underneath the cups turned a deep purple color.

"My heavens," Patti cried when she returned to the room a few minutes later. "You really do have a lot of anger in you. This practice should help draw the hot dark yang energy out of you. It is used extensively in eastern Europe, Asia and parts of the Mediterranean."

Swiftly, she removed each of the cups, explaining that their purpose was to draw toxins in the blood to the skin surface. Once trapped under each cup, these toxins were then driven back into the bloodstream in a concentrated mass when the cups were removed. In this concentrated form, the toxins could more quickly and efficiently be eliminated from the body through the bowels, urine and skin instead of waiting for them to trickle out of the body over time.

"Think of the cups as miniature plungers used to unclog plumbing," she explained with her usual buoyant enthusiasm. "First we suck up the toxins, then when I remove each cup, we flush the toxins out of the body."

Amazingly, the treatment worked. Within minutes, I felt significantly less agitated and deeply relaxed. I left, as I always did when Patti treated me, feeling lighter, brighter and refreshed. Although I could never quite figure out exactly what she did, I could always feel the results. She was a gifted healer.

Jim's description of the effects of prednisone proved accurate. Within hours of taking my first dose, I felt a sharp increase in my appetite, energy and anxiety levels. I also grew sleepless. At 2 or 3 a.m., I would find myself wide awake and feeling like I was going to jump out of my skin. Although prednisone is not an amphetamine, it seemed to produce similar effects. My hands shook and my mind raced. Meditation was the only thing that seemed to help settle me mentally.

My physical coping strategy was different. When we could get out to the hills, I blew off "steroid steam" hiking. The "roids" were amazingly energy producing. Each week, I increased my vertical gain. Within a month, I was hauling myself up several thousand or more vertical feet at a time. At the same time, however, I knew that my strength was temporary and that as soon as I was off steroids, my energy would dissipate. I tried not to think about the crash coming when I headed over that precipice.

The prednisone had the most detrimental effect on my personality and consequently, on my relationship with Cecilia. My actions and moods became wild and unpredictable. I was quick to react angrily, and I found myself constantly agitated and anxious. I worried endlessly about the insignificant. My only sanctuary seemed to be the mountains, but even there, although my anxiety was quelled by exertion, I was still not myself.

One day on a mountain hike, Cecilia said she felt the terrain was too steep for her to comfortably scramble any higher. So while she waited on a safe slope of rock a short distance below the peak, I quickly tagged the top and returned. She had not asked me not to go, but when I got back down to her a few minutes later, she was furious.

"Damn you for leaving me here!" she screamed as frozen tears stuck to her ashen visage. "I've stood by your bedside day in and day out for months and you just left me here on these rocks. I was scared, cold and alone."

I was shocked. Had there been a miscommunication? Perhaps the high exposure had frightened her. The ground was steep, but it was not life-threatening – at least not in my eyes. But my point of view was not the most important one. Hers was.

Judging from the pallid color of her face, she had been badly shaken by something, but by exactly what I did not know. I sensed there was a deeper issue. Sheltering her from the wind, I tried to console her but it was impossible.

Had I made a mistake in going ahead to the top of the peak? Had that impulse been the result of insensitivity, or steroids, or a selfish need to regain lost ground? Both of us had been wrestling with our pasts – Cecilia to let go of hers and me to regain mine.

As we slowly descended in silence, I wondered if our relationship, even our lives, would ever be the same. When we got to the bottom, we tried to talk about what had happened, but it was days before we could. Had I known my departure for the summit would trigger such a forceful reaction, I would never have left her. Obviously, her fear of being abandoned was just as intense as my own fear of dying. But if I died, I would simply move on to another dimension. Cecilia would be left alone with her grief and the reality of trying to make a new life by herself. The stress on her was actually greater than that on me. Both the survivor *and* the caregiver needed care. But because the healthcare system was stretched to the limit treating the survivors, the caregivers' needs were often forgotten. We wondered whether more patients would survive if both caregiver and survivor were treated as one. Their lives were fundamentally intertwined and often stressed to the breaking point.

The next day was Christmas Eve. That helped redirect us to something outside ourselves. We spent the evening at Dale and Cathy's annual Christmas party. Although I was too weak from the hike to stay long, I delighted in listening to our friend, John Clarke, at the piano while Dale and Cathy's seven-year-old daughter Georgia sang her heart out and danced around the Christmas tree. I sat on a chair curled up in a blanket with Cecilia at my side, my bald head adorned with felt moose antlers. In my lap, I cuddled my own personal tin of Cathy's homemade shortbread cookies, surely the best on Earth. I still could taste very little, but a dozen or so of the melt-in-your-mouth biscuits disappeared down my throat in minutes. Steroids or no steroids, I vowed that if I was going to turn into the Goodyear blimp, at least I was going to do it in style.

Scrooge may have spurned the ghost of Christmas Past and feared the ghost of Christmas Future, but Cecilia and I awoke on Christmas morning giving thanks for Christmas Present. We were alive and together, and like Tiny Tim, a Higher Power had definitely blessed us, every one.

As Cecilia and I spooned on the sofa beside our little Christmas tree that morning, I remembered Charlie Brown's forlorn little equivalent. I pictured it, bent over by the weight of a single fragile bulb, but wrapped warmly in a blanket of love. Even as it appeared weak and frail, it was still standing, as were we.

The moment filled us with more than joy. It filled us with gratitude.

CHAPTER 34

Cecilia

PEAK

STRESS

Life together is starting to take on new shape. I am beginning to know when to pull back from my caregiving so Alan doesn't feel smothered. Sometimes I feel like an adolescent again, uncertain of who I am or where I fit in.

10th Tool for *Caregivers*
Support, Don't Smother

It's a cool and windy December day. Alan has a newfound energy called prednisone. It is a strong medication that keeps the Graft Versus Host Disease in check. With Alan's new energy has come a resurgence of his desire for life as it was before leukemia. He wants to get back to the mountains and I fully support him in this. We've decided to take a hike up one of the nearby peaks in Canmore. I begin to prepare our lunch while Alan starts gathering hiking boots and the other gear for the day.

We drive west from Calgary a little over an hour, through the prairies, towards the mountains. Again, I feel liberated from the confinement of the apartment and the hospital. With vast stretches of open land just outside the city, I want to keep driving as far as possible. The spaciousness of it all is so much more evident to me now. We drive past fields with bales of hay cast golden by the sunlight. There's little snow.

When we park at the trailhead, Alan pops out of the car like a frisky dog at his favorite park. This is Alan's territory. The Rockies are majestic as always. Standing at the base of the mountain, I take in the immeasurable beauty around us.

Although I lived the majority of my life in New Orleans – below sea level – I have always had an affinity for mountains. Each Mardi Gras, I would escape the raucous partying and travel to Colorado to ski hard for five days and nights. I always returned exhausted but exhilarated from the experience. The Canadian Rockies are no different. I've had to learn to pace myself while adjusting to the altitude. The elevation taxes my energy and I can easily end up gasping for air.

Prednisone-fueled Alan starts out on the trail. I find myself rushing to catch up. My fitness is at an all-time low, and this is a brisker pace than our previous hikes. Since August, exercise has been one of those things I "should do for myself." Doing something for myself, though, took too much energy, energy I didn't have. Most days I would forego the "something for me" to check off another "to do" item on my list. There would be time for me later, I thought.

Swift pace or not, it's always great to be back on a mountain trail. The quiet sounds of the forest are what I notice first. No more static-filled announcements over the hospital intercom system. No I.V. alarms going off to alert the nurses the infusion of chemotherapy has ended. The only sound is the soft rush of the wind blowing through the trees.

I find myself lagging behind Alan up the mountain. I watch as his boundless energy carries him up the trail with little effort. We're on a fairly straightforward hike with only the occasional tree root or boulder to traverse. Otherwise, it's a well-defined trail for most of the way up. I can feel the strain in my calves, a by-product of spending too much time sitting lately. But I continue on, savoring the scent of pine and spruce in the air.

After a couple of hours of hiking, we break above the tree line. A burst of cold air hits my face and slaps me to attention. After some steep hiking, we come to an exposed area below the summit. This is where the trail ends. The last one hundred and fifty feet or so to the top require some knowledge of hand-over-hand scrambling on all fours. It also requires more concentration. At this point in my life, I have little of either. I'm outside my comfort zone. Unsure of my next move, I lose my footing and slide backwards. Alan reaches to take my hand.

"Are you all right?" he asks.

I cannot answer.

Judging I'm safe, Alan says, "Okay, wait here. I'll be to the summit and back in a few minutes."

He may think I'm safe, but I don't feel that way. As soon as he leaves, I am gripped by fear. Every part of my body clings to the icy-cold, unforgiving rock. I feel vulnerable and exposed, both physically and psychologically. A few tears start to slide down my face. Then, as if my eyes are too tired to hold back the floodwaters, a river of tears begins to flow. Grief takes hold and I can't stop it. My fear of abandonment overwhelms me. The sound of my sobbing is muffled by the howling wind. No one can hear me cry – for this I am grateful. In a way, it feels good to release the anger and frustration I've been feeling for so long.

After about ten minutes, Alan returns, triumphant at having reached the summit. With his help, I'm able to free my death grip and slowly move down to a flatter spot.

Eventually, we start the long hike back down. On so many of our previous hikes, descent was a time for laughter and celebration. Today, we move in silence. I have nothing left for merriment. I'm too wrapped in grief to feel any joy.

Part of me understands Alan's intense need to achieve the summit, but the more immediate part of me is awash in sadness. It feels like yet another test of our relationship. I cannot celebrate and he cannot grieve.

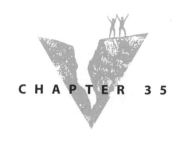

CHAPTER 35

Alan
WALKING

"Do not go where the path may lead; go instead where there is no path and leave a trail."

– Ralph Waldo Emerson,
American Philosopher and Writer

We awoke on New Year's Day with a feeling of triumph.

"Goodbye leukemia, hello life!" I shrieked as Cecilia looked on wide-eyed from beneath the blankets. For the first time in months, I had slept solidly through the night. It was a good start to a new year, and we were ready to embrace it. This was going to be our year. This was going to be the year we came back to life.

But it would be a slow journey. Three days into January, almost halfway to the important hundred-day milestone, I exploded in a rage while trying to pump up a bicycle tire. When I was unable to get the pump to work, I bludgeoned it to pieces. Cecilia left me alone to work it out.

The next day I called Karen Sabo, one of the nurses at the Bone Marrow Transplant Clinic.

"If you don't get me off these steroids soon, I'm either going to turn into the Pillsbury Doughboy, kill someone or kill myself," I blasted. "Please get me off this stuff – now!"

There was silence on the other end of the line. I can only imagine what she must have been thinking. How *do* you placate a roaring tiger?

"Are there any other symptoms you may be experiencing?" she inquired calmly, maintaining her composure.

"I think that's enough, don't you?" I continued, bristling. "I feel like I'm going to jump out of my skin. I'm totally wired, my hands are shaking, I can't focus mentally, and physically, I can't seem to slow down. I'm like a rat on an exercise wheel except that at least the rat can control how fast he's running. How long is it going to take to get me off this?"

"That's a very good question, Alan, and we need to approach it very carefully," she continued, showing remarkable self-control. "If we take you off the steroids too suddenly, you could really experience complications from withdrawal. Or the Graft Versus Host Disease could return. So if we do decide to take you off the medication, we'll need to take you down in slow easy steps. I'll talk to one of the docs and see what's best."

What was best, it was determined, was to put me on yet another drug, this time a mild tranquilizer to calm me down while I was tapered off the prednisone.

On January 4, my parents came to visit. It was tremendous to see them both again, especially my father, Peter, whom I had not seen since before my diagnosis. During my treatment, he had chosen to stay in Ottawa and cheer me on by telephone. He would analyze information he received during our phone conversations and when we next spoke, suggest possible courses of action. At other times, he just listened intently, took notes (as did my mother) and provided unconditional love and support. But if I had ever needed him to be physically there for me, just like my mother, he would have been there in an instant.

Together, we toured the hospital and I introduced them to the nurses and staff at the Bone Marrow Transplant Clinic. It was located across the hall from where Cecilia and I had received my diagnosis from Dr. Poon. I thought it would be memorable if my parents could meet him, so on the spur of the moment, I asked if he might be able to squeeze in a visit. He surprised me not only by showing up on very short notice, but also by posing for photographs with us.

That evening Dr. Poon went home with a headache, feeling feverish. He later collapsed and was rushed unconscious by ambulance to the Emergency Room of Foothills where he stopped breathing and almost died. Only quick action on the part of the Emergency Room staff saved his life. It was later determined he had a serious blood infection called septicemia and had gone into shock. To his complete amazement, he awoke from a coma in the Intensive Care Unit the next morning. He was hooked up to a ventilator, with tubes coming out of all orifices, peering into the bloodshot eyes of his wife, daughter and son. They had kept vigil all night by his bedside. Somehow, he had come in contact with a particularly virulent strain of E. coli bacteria, perhaps through one of his patients during a prostate biopsy the previous day. At first, it was resistant to modern antibiotics, but when an older antibiotic was tried, it succumbed and Dr. Poon recovered.

I did not learn of his brush with death until a week later when during a routine visit to the hospital for a blood test, I bumped into him wearing a hospital gown, in a wheelchair, on his way to get an ultrasound test. He had been released from ICU to a regular ward the night before and was already up and around on his own.

"That was damned close," he said pensively. "Maybe a half breadth of a hair away and very humbling. I now have a much better appreciation for what patients go through when they're sick and it will make me a better doctor. I am very thankful indeed that I am around and able to talk to you today. Every day, as you know, is a bonus."

Three days later, the resilient doctor-turned-patient was home to celebrate his fifty-ninth birthday.

After the huge physical and psychological build-up to transplant, I now found myself waking up to a new world, discovering what my new life would be like. For the most part, although I was supremely grateful to be alive, I did not like what I saw. I continued to be fearful that my fatigue would return as soon as I went off prednisone and that I might never again be able to fully engage in life as I once had. Where I had once run easily along the bicycle paths beside the Bow River, I was now lucky just to walk. If I tried to jog, I became exhausted very quickly. It was a constant battle not to become demoralized and lament that which I had lost, rather than celebrate that which I still had. The practice of gratitude required as much mental discipline as physical training did.

"I am now realizing just how far I have to go to come back," I wrote in my diary one day in late January. "This is going to be a long road and I'm looking down a long pipe. I wonder if I'll ever be back to a physical fraction of what I was before or whether that part of my life is gone forever now and I just have to grieve the loss and adjust as best I can. Physically, I feel as if I've been cut in half. I am no longer a high performance athlete. Now I am an average person, alive, yes, but average."

Cecilia watched me grapple with this adjustment. It must have been hard for her, but as usual she remained optimistic.

"You will rebuild yourself just like you rebuilt yourself after each Everest expedition," she told me repeatedly. "It's not a matter of *if*, it's a matter of *when*."

"You don't understand," I countered. "It *is* a matter of if. No one to the best of my knowledge has ever been able to rebuild themselves to an elite level of fitness after a blood transplant for leukemia. We're breaking new ground."

"Great," she said confidently, "because I can think of no better person to do it than you. Go ahead. Break the trail. I'm right behind you."

As soon as she said that, a light turned on inside my head. I thought of the historic moment on May 29, 1953 when Edmund Hillary and Sherpa Tenzing Norgay had approached the knife-edged ridge between the south summit of Everest and the base of what is now called The Hillary Step, a rock step a short distance down from the top of the world. As their heads scraped the sky at over 28,500 feet, they were faced with a terrifying prospect. On one side of the ridge was a ghastly six thousand foot drop into

Nepal. On the other was an equally nerve-wracking eight thousand foot drop into Tibet. In places, the ridge was only one foot wide. And no one in the history of the world had ever set foot there.

While our challenge was hardly the same in magnitude or significance, Cecilia had hit upon something very important. Unknowingly, she had stimulated my imagination. My best performances as a gymnast had always been preceded by my strongest visualizations of them. So now, even while I was physically weak, there was nothing to stop me from imagining myself hiking smoothly up mountains or pedaling strongly up a hill on a mountain bike. It seemed that I could do these activities with the help of steroids. But could I do them without steroids? This was where I needed to clear another hurdle.

I had imagined for years what it would look like and feel like to stand on the summit of Everest on a beautiful, calm, blue-sky day. Then on May 23, 1997, that is exactly what had happened. Now I imagined myself back to full fitness, full strength and a full life. I would point myself up the slope and take the first step.

More important for me than this visualization, however, was Cecilia's idea of turning my cancer experience into a comeback that might assist others. I pulled out Lance Armstrong's book and noticed with interest that his oncologist had referred to cancer as "The Tour de France of Illnesses." If I could come back from my own Everest of Illnesses, perhaps, like Lance, I could help others overcome their own serious setbacks. I liked the idea of breaking trail for others, pioneering a new route up a very big, frightening and dangerous mountain. In fact, it excited me more than doing it only for myself. For the first time in my illness, I understood that cancer, or more accurately, a climb back from this kind of cancer and its debilitating treatment could be "the ultimate adventure" – the very words that had been used for decades to describe the earliest ascents of Everest. I took hold of this idea and when I did, it began to transform the way I looked at my illness. It became more than exciting to me. It became inspirational.

Two days before my final bone marrow biopsy, on February 5, I celebrated my forty-third birthday. Cecilia surprised me by whisking me away to a secluded log cabin in the foothills. We slept late, went for a short walk and just relaxed. It was great to be out of the apartment and back in the hills again.

Dr. Christian Fibich performed the final bone marrow biopsy. At thirty-five, he was a bright and enthusiastic oncologist on a fellowship from Germany. Jim Russell continued to oversee my treatment, but Christian was now responsible for my follow-up care in the outpatient clinic. Gradually, Cecilia and I were being given more freedom.

I liked Christian very much. He weight trained, and was strong and muscular. His arms and chest looked especially powerful and he had calluses on the palms of his hands and fingertips that had the look and feel of shoe leather. They reminded me of Laurie Skreslet's. Although Christian looked almost too young to be a doctor, he carried himself with confidence. It was obvious he was being groomed for something greater. He had been assigned many of Dr. Russell's patients, so clearly, Jim had confidence in him. That was all the endorsement I needed.

"I've been given the okay from Dr. Russell to use an ice screw to perform the biopsy," Christian said in his German accent.

We burst into laughter. I wondered how Christian could possibly know what an ice screw was, and just as importantly, that it was many times the diameter of a bone marrow biopsy needle.

The young German, it turned out, was a very experienced rock climber capable of scaling extreme routes. He had climbed extensively worldwide and trained whenever he could.

What were the chances of my oncologist being a climber? And what were the chances he would understand completely what it was like to take a long fall? Again I felt like someone was sending me a message that everything was going to be okay. If I would just relax, stop worrying and have a little faith, things would work out.

On February 14, Valentine's Day, our hope was reborn. My bone marrow biopsy results came back clear. There was no evidence of leukemia at all.

Cecilia and I jumped for joy, high-fiving and laughing and twirling each other around. We were euphoric.

"These results are as good as they get," Christian declared. "You're in complete remission. Let's book you in to have your central line removed."

Cecilia and I hit the roof again. We cheered until the tears rolled down our faces. We were going to be liberated from the line! We were going to lose that albatross around my neck, the constant reminder that I was sick! Baby fuzz was starting to reappear on my bald head, and soon I might be able to swim again too. That would be glorious! That would be magnificent! I could float face down in a pool. I could put my head under water in the bathtub!

Three days later, Christian removed my central line. It took him quite a bit of digging with a scalpel to get it out of my chest. It was as if my body knew it was a lifeline. But with some help from Dr. Chaudry, Christian succeeded. Finally, the line slipped from my chest. Christian put in a few simple stitches and the deed was done.

"There now," he said triumphantly. "No more plastic in your pecs, Alan. You're a free man."

Tilting my chest to one side to protect the stitches, I gave him a hug.

"Thank you, Christian!" I babbled. "Bless you, bless you, bless you."

"It was nothing," he demurred, smiling.

Of course it was something. It was something very big. And everyone knew it, especially us.

"Good riddance chemotherapy, blood draws and immunity in a bag," Cecilia said, beaming. "We're one step closer to a normal life."

A little over a week later, on February 23, Cecilia and I celebrated Day 100. We had been invited to a fundraising dinner that evening for the Canadian Cancer Society. So we packed up the cardboard cutout of Bolek's medical mountain, carried it into the ballroom of Calgary's Fairmont Palliser Hotel and carefully placed it on an easel beside the podium. Then, sporting tiny patches of hair and the best rented tux I could afford, I swallowed my pride and when called upon, stepped up to the microphone before four hundred people. Cecilia and I had made sure we had personally invited Bolek and his wife, Halina, to hear what I had to say.

The room, which had been abuzz with laughter and conversation, suddenly went silent.

I started by talking about the Sherpas. I spoke about the ones who had greeted me on Everest when I had returned from the summit to base camp. Each of them had presented me with a special silk scarf. These had been blessed by the local lama and had strong spiritual meaning.

Slowly, I held up one of the scarves. Then, after presenting Bolek's cardboard creation and introducing him, I asked him to come forward.

"Before my transplant, I used to think that the Sherpas only existed in Nepal," I explained as he made his way to the stage. "I was wrong. I met dozens of them on my medical mountain. Bolek has the heart and soul of a Sherpa."

The crowd rose to its feet in vigorous applause. As reverently as I could, I reached up and placed the scarf around Bolek's neck. Then I gave him a huge hug like the one Laurie Skreslet had given to me that day in the hospital so many months before. Our souls met.

"Bolek works as a personal care assistant," I concluded, "but that's not how I know him and that's not how he is known by the thousands of patients whose lives he has positively affected through his work. We not only call him a Sherpa. We call him a hero."

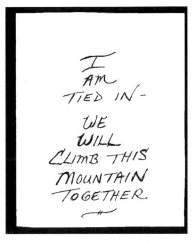

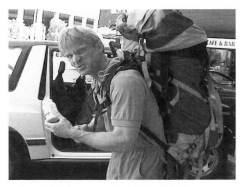

23. Departing for Inner Everest Base Camp: The Medical Mountain Expedition leaves from downtown Calgary. The thought of weeks of hospital food made Alan grimace.

Alan: *"It was like sitting on the edge of a glacial crevasse with the frigid air blowing up at me from the icy abyss below. It chilled me deeply."*

Photo Credit: Cecilia Hobson

22. Ten Courageous Words: Cecilia's note to Alan after the diagnosis.

Alan: *"This was love -- quiet, solid, unshakable -- the stuff of dreams, the stuff you only come across once in a lifetime if you are lucky and I had stumbled upon a mother lode. In its simplicity and purity, it went far beyond romance. It was absolute and powerful."*

Photo Credit: Cecilia Hobson

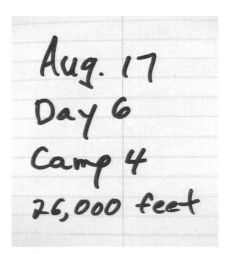

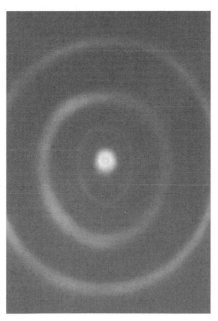

24. Transforming the Unknown into the Known: One of the notes Cecilia posted on the door of Alan's hospital room during chemotherapy.

Alan: *"The closer we got to the end of the chemotherapy cycle, the worse I was likely to feel. In fact, I felt exactly the way I did as I got closer to the summit of Everest. Headaches were common. So was acute fatigue, nausea, vomiting and insomnia. I tried to imagine each round of chemotherapy like a summit bid on Everest."*

Photo Credit: Cecilia Hobson

25. A Point of Peace: The picture on which Alan focused his mind during open eye meditation.

Alan: *"I disappeared within myself. Then I let myself become completely calm, as if I was looking over a beautiful vista on a clear, blue-sky day. It made me feel warm and safe."*

Photo Credit: Brahma Kumaris World Spiritual University, London

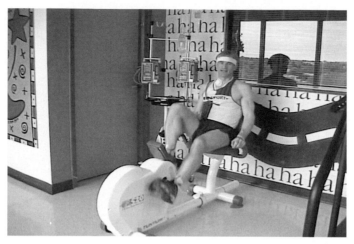

26. Pedaling for His Life: Alan rides the stationary bike on the Foothills Medical Centre's Unit 57 cancer ward during chemotherapy.

Cecilia: *"Off to one end of the ward, there is a sitting area with a lone stationary bike and treadmill. Unlike the scene in a gym, there is no humming of equipment beneath the beat of music, no televisions hanging from the ceilings, no other sweaty bodies synchronized in movement in a row of treadmills, but the picture of Alan on the stationary bike is the same to me."*

Photo Credit: Cecilia Hobson

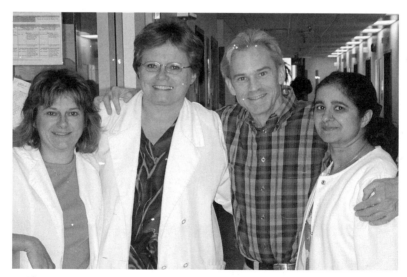

27. The Front Lines: Alan with (L-R) nurse Carol Spitzer, Unit 57 patient care manager Marilyn Bouchard, and nurse Inderjit "Digit" Khaira, members of the outstanding staff on the Foothills Medical Centre's Unit 57.

Alan: *"There was a desire among the staff to perform at their peak so that in the end, whatever the outcome, there would be no dishonor. I liked that about 57. There was a truthfulness to the place."*

Photo Credit: Cecilia Hobson

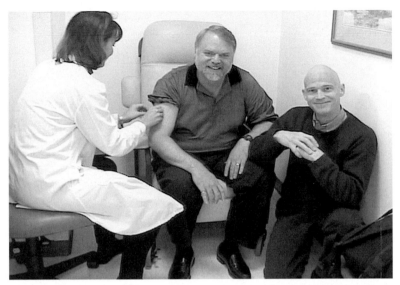

28. Injection of Hope: Alan kneels as nurse Naree Ager of the Foothills Medical Centre's Bone Marrow Transplant Clinic gives Eric the all-important injection of the Amgen drug, NEUPOGEN. It stimulated the production of adult blood stem cells and made the transplant possible.

Alan: *"'They can't take my stem cells out of you if the transplant doesn't work, can they?' Eric asked moments before the transplant. 'No,' said acute care nurse Rita Dillabough as she prepared one of the bags of Eric's adult blood stem cells for infusion, 'but it'll work.' 'It will work,' Eric echoed."*

Photo Credit: Cecilia Hobson

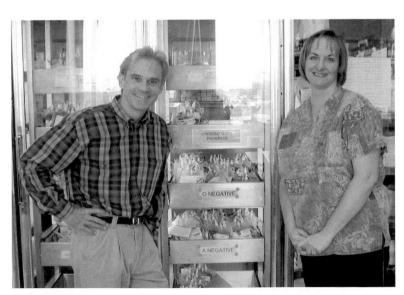

29. Cool Compassion: Alan with medical laboratory technologist, Susan Berrigan, before the precious blood bank refrigerator she oversaw at Foothills Medical Centre.

Alan: *"I would receive regular transfusions from completely anonymous donors to whose compassion and generosity I owe my life."*

Photo Credit: Cecilia Hobson

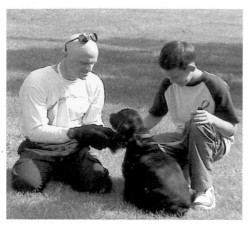

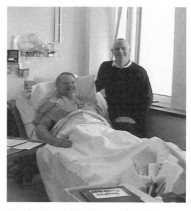

30. A Bald Man's Best Friend: Alan with the near-blind Cocker Spaniel, Oreo, and Garret Dillabough, acute care nurse Rita Dillabough's son.

Cecilia: *"It is as if Oreo knows Alan needs her love, and she gives it openly. I watch with a smile on my face and a glow in my heart as a bond forms between dog and man that transcends most human connections."*

Photo Credit: Cecilia Hobson

31. Liquid Gold: As Alan stands at his bedside, Eric donates his adult blood stem cells at the Apherisis Unit of the Foothills Medical Centre. Eric is hooked up to a centrifuge on his right (out of view) which spins off the adult stem cells from his blood.

Alan: *"While Eric joked with the nurses, I watched with excitement as he donated about two hundred million of his adult blood stem cells, roughly the volume of a couple of cups of coffee."*

Photo Credit: Cecilia Hobson

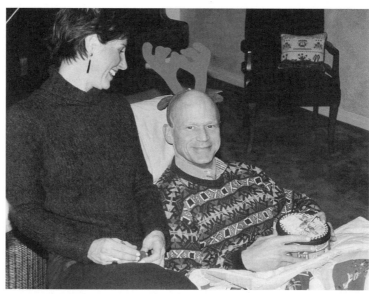

32. The Gift of Christmas Present: Christmas Eve at Dale and Cathy Ens' home six weeks after the transplant.

Alan: *"In my lap, I cuddled my own personal tin of Cathy's homemade shortbread cookies, surely the best on Earth. I ate a dozen or so in minutes. If I was going to turn into the Goodyear blimp, at least I was going to do it in style."*

Photo Credit: Cathy Ens

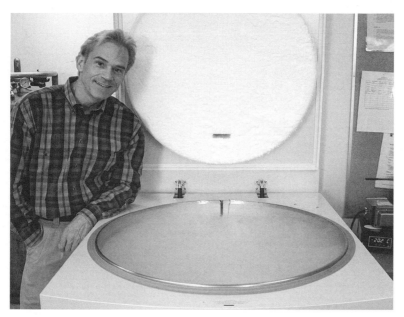

33. Frozen Potential: Alan and the cryofreezer in which three small bags of Eric's adult blood stem cells were stored at minus 180 degrees [C] in liquid nitrogen. The vapors are the result of the nitrogen boiling at room temperature.

Alan: *"'That's a funky effect,' I said motioning towards the basin. 'It looks like a cross between a magic show and a science experiment.'"*

Photo Credit: Cecilia Hobson

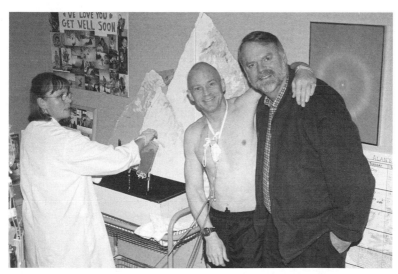

34. Blood Brothers: Alan and Eric minutes before the transplant. Technician Judy Ranson thaws the first bag of Eric's adult blood stem cells to prepare them for infusion.

Alan: *"The bags were so small compared to the power they held. 'A new life is going to come out of those little things?' I wondered to myself. It was unbelievable."*

Photo Credit: ABL Imaging

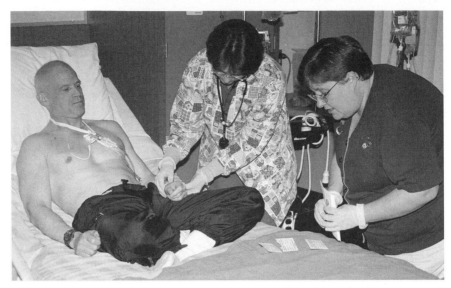

35. Moment of Truth: The transplant begins. Acute care nurses Rita Dillabough (center) and Kim Stoop cross-check Alan's patient number with the number on the tags from Eric's adult blood stem cells.

Cecilia: *"The energy in the room on transplant day is electrifying. The adrenalin is flowing through my veins as if I am under attack. In a way I am. There is so much riding on this day…"*

Photo Credit: ABL Imaging

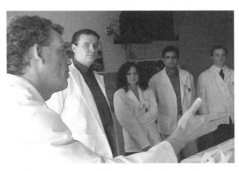

36. Sharing the Knowledge: One of Alan's oncologists, Dr. Chris Brown, teaching a group of medical students at Alan's bedside. Chris is one of Canada's leading leukemia researchers and a strong advocate of physical activity in cancer prevention and recovery.

Alan: *"Outside each room, the resident, attending physician, charge nurse and sometimes a few medical students discussed the condition of the patient they were about to visit. Whenever I heard that 'the pack' was starting its way down my wing of the ward, I would make sure to stay close to my room. The result of rounds often determined if I could go home on a day or overnight pass."*

Photo Credit: Cecilia Hobson

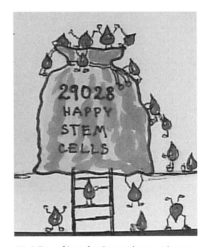

37. A Bag of Laughs: Personal care assistant Bolek Babiarz's drawing of a bag of 29,028 happy adult blood stem cells -- one for every foot that Mt. Everest is tall.

Alan: *"My first visitor on transplant day was Bolek. He broke the tension by pulling out a pen, walking up to my daily blood cell count calendar and creating a delightful drawing of adult blood stem cells. He called them my 'Happy Cells.' Within minutes, he had me feeling happy too."*

Drawing by: Bolek Babiarz

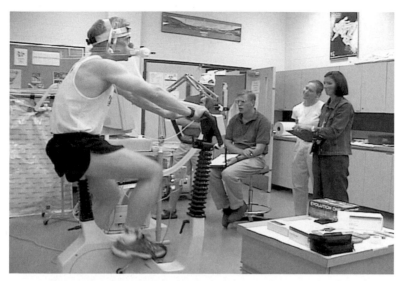

38. One of the Keys to Overcoming Chronic Fatigue? Alan on the bike at the University of Calgary during the early days of the Survivor Fatigue Study that led to *The Climb Back from Cancer Protocol*. L – R: Alan's personal training coach, Cal Zaryski (wearing white baseball hat behind equipment); Olympic exercise physiologist, Dr. David Smith (seated with clipboard); and associates Jodi Hawley and Maura Hooper.

Alan: *"Astonishingly, the survivors in our study increased their energy levels by an average of fifty percent to match those experienced by adults in the general population. Mood disturbances such as depression, anxiety and anger decreased by sixty-five percent, and participants reported more vigor and less difficulty with memory and decision-making. This is the goal that now drives Cecilia and me: to instill this hope in more and more people."*

Photo Credit: Cecilia Hobson

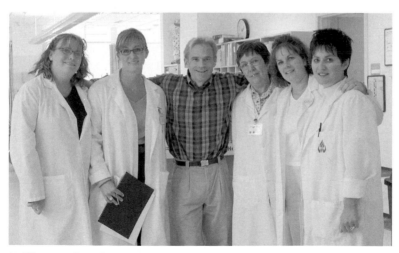

39. Lifesavers: Alan with (L-R) nurses Bonnie McMillan, Krista MacAlister, Linda Hassman, Heather Omilon and Karen Sabo of the Foothills Medical Centre's Bone Marrow Transplant Clinic.

Alan: *"After weeks on the steroid prednisone, I called Karen Sabo. 'If you don't get me off these steroids soon, I'm either going to turn into the Pillsbury Doughboy, kill someone or kill myself,' I blasted. 'Get me off this stuff – now!'"*

Photo Credit: Cecilia Hobson

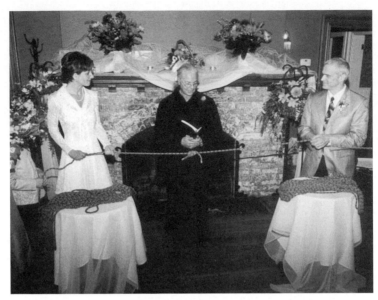

40. A Triumph of Love over Adversity: With Marriage Commissioner, Nomi Whalen, we literally tie the knot with two climbing ropes.

Cecilia: *"As Alan pulls his rope and I pull mine, I gaze into his eyes. At the moment the two knots join into one, my heart jumps and our new beginning takes hold, one radiant with hope."*

Photo Credit: Bruce Kirkby

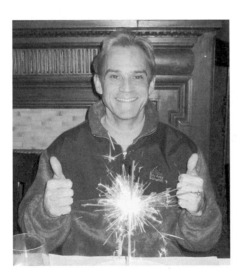

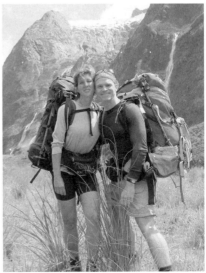

41. A Sparkling Victory: Alan's surprise 1st re-birthday party.

Alan: *"As everyone sang 'Happy 1st Re-Birthday,' I watched in wonder as a single sparkler candle burned its way slowly down toward the inch-thick icing on my chocolate birthday cake. Every day from here on would be like the icing on that cake."*

Photo Credit: Cecilia Hobson

42. A Team Triumph: Our honeymoon in New Zealand. Delayed by cancer, but never cancelled.

"Now you are two people but with one path before you. May your days be good and long upon this earth." – Apache Blessing

Photo Credit: Alan and Cecilia Hobson

CHAPTER 36

Cecilia
VICTORIOUS
LOVE

Today I'm remembering last winter, a beautiful Rocky Mountain day with fresh snow, sunshine and little wind. It was Sunday, February 13, six months before Alan's diagnosis. He was leaving the next day for a speaking engagement. We would not be together for Valentine's Day, so to celebrate early we decided to spend the weekend hiking near Banff.

That morning, while we were sitting next to a roaring fire in a restaurant, Alan said he would pop out to the national park office to check the weather forecast for the day. I thought it wasn't necessary because he had checked it earlier that morning. But I knew how thorough Alan was, and it was not unusual for him to do a second or third check of anything.

I enjoyed every minute of the snowshoe hike. Feeling the energy of the mountains, I kept my pace steady up the steep slope to a natural amphitheater surrounded by sheer rock faces. The trees gave way to the most beautiful snow-covered carpet. It was a perfect setting in which to stop for a bite to eat. We took off our packs and sat down to take in the splendor. Alan started digging into his backpack – I thought to find his heavy parka – but to my surprise, he pulled out a long cardboard box with a card attached. I opened it, and the words filled me with warmth like the sweetest cup of hot apple cider. The opening line read, "Thank you for making every day Valentine's Day when we are together."

In the box was a bouquet of a dozen long-stemmed red roses. He had taken such care to ensure they would retain their beauty through the two-hour hike in freezing temperatures. The box was filled with several hand-warmer packets that produced heat to protect the blooms. He hadn't gone to the park office for weather information that morning – he'd gone to pick up roses!

Slowly, he picked up one of the roses, got down on one knee, handed me the rose and asked, "Will you marry me?" I was overwhelmed with emotion. The combination of the altitude and my racing heart left me weak in the knees. I responded, "You know my answer is yes."

In the eight months I have been caring for Alan, we never knew if our wedding day would ever come. Today, a little over a year after he proposed, that day has finally arrived.

My dream, fueled by fond memories of the New Orleans springtime, has always been a spring wedding outdoors. I had wanted a trellis for Alan and me to walk through. The classical arch is a centuries-old symbol of passage from one space to another and the transition of time. It marks entrances to special places and suggests new beginnings. With all my heart, I want our marriage to transcend the cancer experience. Hand in hand, we will enter a special new place together. Unfortunately, because of the weather, an outdoor trellis isn't practical. But we will walk through one in our minds and hearts; we are set on a fresh beginning.

It is the morning of March 22, one day into spring on the calendar, and it's snowing. In the Canadian Rockies, March is still winter and spring weather is months away. The Ranche Restaurant is nestled in Fish Creek Provincial Park south of Calgary. The building was constructed in 1896 and has been fully restored to maintain the romance of the West. With the arrival of snow, our planned outdoor gathering has been moved indoors. Our lounge-style room has comfortable couches and chairs, a wood-burning fireplace and a bay window. It feels like we have stepped back in time, back to the days when this historic house was one of southern Alberta's grandest private residences. There is already a brilliant fire burning in the hundred-year-old fireplace. The flames seem to dance for joy in anticipation of our impending nuptials.

Because we want the simplest of ceremonies, we don't have all our friends and family with us in person, but we feel their presence. The wedding party consists of dear friends. Dale is best man and his wife, Cathy, is matron of honor. Their daughter, Georgia, is our flower girl and vocalist. Bruce Kirkby, one of Alan's friends and fellow adventurers is our photographer, and his girlfriend, Christine, is operating the video camera. Nomi Whalen, our Marriage Commissioner, presides over the ceremony.

The smell of hickory and the crackle of the fire create the perfect setting. Alan and I stand facing one another in front of the fireplace, its mantle adorned with flowers, as Nomi begins the ceremony. I look at him with girlish rapture. His hair is just beginning to grow back and he looks so handsome in his suit jacket. As Alan begins to affirm his vows, I feel a joy and peace within me that I haven't felt since he was diagnosed. His voice is calm and clear as he speaks the words, "I will stand by your side even when we grow old." Growing old together is something every young couple believes will happen. I do not have the luxury of being so naïve. The words hang in the air. I find myself picturing us still hiking in our eighties. I hold back tears at the possibility of such a dream coming true.

We want our wedding rings to be special, a sign of the strength of our bond. We want them made in the likeness of a grapevine knot. In climbing, the grapevine knot is often used to tie two pieces of rope together so climbers can lower themselves safely to the ground. What makes the knot unique is that it actually consists of two separate knots that when pulled together become one. Because our rings aren't ready, we have decided to use the next best thing – climbing rope itself. This evening, we literally and figuratively tie the knot.

"With the pulling of these ropes, I promise to give to you the truth, my trust, my support, my respect and my love," we both say. As Alan pulls his rope and I pull mine, I gaze into his eyes. Our knots move closer to becoming one. I can hear Nomi saying, "Let the joining of these two knots be symbolic of the joining of your two souls." At the moment the two knots join into one, my heart jumps and our new beginning takes hold.

Nomi reads an Apache blessing:

Now there is no rain
For each of you will be shelter for the other.
Now there is no cold
For each of you will be warmth for the other.
Now there is no loneliness
For each of you will be companion to the other.
Now you are two people
But with one path before you.
Go now to your dwelling
To enter into the days of your life together.
And may your days be good and long
Upon this earth.

I silently repeat to myself, *"And may your days be good and long upon this earth."* We kiss. Georgia's angelic voice takes me to a place over the rainbow "where troubles melt like lemon drops and dreams you dare to dream really do come true." Tears of joy stream down my face. The magical lyrics take me to a new place – somewhere far from hospitals and radiant with hope.

CHAPTER 37

Alan
RUNNING

My mission was to overcome my latest illness and get back in the game. Now I really had to deliver – to the best of my ability, for better or for worse, summit or no summit.

– From Everest to Enlightenment

A few days after honoring Bolek, I took my first swim. My friend, Hal Kuntze, happened to be in the pool training.

"Hobson!" he cried. "This is your first swim since your transplant, isn't it?"

"You betcha!" Cecilia replied as she videotaped the exchange. "Face down in the water is sure gonna beat face down in a hospital bed."

"Good on ya," Hal said, cheering. "You guys are an awesome team."

Slowly, I slipped into the pool. It was *cold*. Instantly I started to shiver.

I put my face into the water. I had dreamed of this moment for months. Now at last it was here. Now at last I could be weightless.

I pushed off from the wall and glided face down. It was divine. Even if I was shivering, it felt like I was slipping back into an old comfortable sock.

I swam only a few lengths before I got too cold to continue, but it was enough to assure me I could still swim. That part of me was still there. It would take months and years to build myself back, but for the first time it didn't matter how long I swam or even how far. It was enough just to experience it. My joy, like my immersion, was total.

The next phase in my recovery followed soon after. In early March, I began feeling inexplicably anxious, increasingly depressed and fearful of the future. In my diary I wrote:

> We've cleared the first hundred days and now we're faced with the next hundred days or the next thousand days or however many days it is. What am I to do now with whatever time I have left? Is it best to just play for three years until I can be more confident I'll survive? Is that when my life can begin again? Should I just try to go back to speaking, but do fewer presentations? Or should I stop speaking altogether, find a place in the mountains and spend the rest of my days adventuring for as long as the money lasts? These are the questions rolling around in my head. But in addition to the trauma I've just come through, for some reason I've got the shakes. The prednisone is finished, so it's not that. It's something else…. It's by far the most difficult part of my recovery so far because it's indefinable. I can't seem to figure out the source of the anxiety or what I should do about it.

We had come through treatment and transplant. My immune system was rebuilding itself. So was my blood. Now I could swim again. I had every reason to celebrate, but that is not how I felt. I felt sad and anxious and blue, sometimes even a bit black. What was going on? Was I losing my mind? How come I did not feel happy about being alive?

Unable to understand why, Cecilia and I reported to Helen MacRae.

"This is called survivor grief," she said. "I see it often in those who come through treatment. It is one of the most trying parts of convalescence."

"But why would I be anxious now?" I asked. "We've come through chemo, I've had my transplant, and now we have the rest of our lives to look forward to for as long as the rest of our lives happens to be."

"Well, while you were undergoing treatment you were entirely focused on getting better," she explained. "Now you're starting to realize just how close you actually came to dying. I'm not saying this enterprise is over, because it's not. You know the mortality rate in the first three years as much as I do. Think of it like crossing a very deep crevasse on a ladder that bridges the gap from one side to the other. When do you shake the most – at the beginning, while you're actually making your way across or when you get to the other side?"

"Definitely when you get to the other side," I replied.

"There you go," she confirmed. "This is no different. Think about it."

We did, but it did not seem to help. The anxiety and depression were like a cloud parked over me and it refused to budge. It went everywhere I went because it was in my head and heart. I felt like there was a hole in my soul and somehow I was bleeding through it. I could not afford to lose any more precious blood. I wanted the bleeding to stop. I was grieving the loss of a part of my life I might never regain – my complete physical self. And I was therefore uncertain about what kind of a future I would have. I knew the around-the-world solo ocean sailor, John Hughes, in *One Step Beyond*, would be able to relate. He had somehow survived a dismasting in a terrible storm 1,800 miles from land and realized that while there was often a calm before a storm, there were sometimes the doldrums after it.

"Gone was the victory of having survived," he had said. "What replaced it was an overwhelming cloud of despair, depression and utter solitude…The thought of not completing the race started to depress me so badly that I began to see why people commit suicide."

I was not suicidal, but the idea had crossed my mind. Sometimes, it did not seem like I had much to live for. One day dragged into the next.

Desperate for some relief, I consulted a psychiatrist. He prescribed the antidepressant, Wellbutrin, a medication he was studying to counteract fatigue as well as depression. It made a big difference. Within days, my mental state improved and although I continued to experience anxiety, my gloomy moments were not nearly as dark, long or frequent.

Swimming also helped. Several times a week, I followed a program called "Total Immersion." It was designed to teach you to swim like a fish by reducing your drag through the water. For me, it did more. I would float face down, face up and on my side, kicking my way slowly and silently from one end of the pool to the other, trying to make peace with the water and somehow with myself. I had never been without a significant and tangible goal in my life before. My life, as well as my body, was suspended. What I found, however, was that as I swam, I began to slip into a kind of meditation. With every length of the pool, I fell further and further into a state of relaxation, and unbeknownst to me, revitalization.

This silent process was imperceptible to others and even to me. My goal became only to be in the pool, not to turn it into an athletic event. I forgot about distance, lengths, time or speed. I focused on training my mind as well as my body to rest and be free. I began to connect with the water in a way I never had before. No longer was I fighting it or life. Now I began flowing through it.

I had moved past transplant and embarked on my climb back. If I lived to see five years, the doctors would call it a cure. That is when I hoped to be able to say I had my life back, whatever its form.

Over time, one thing became clear. Cecilia and I could finally get married. We had waited long enough. The treatment, transplant and recovery had taken a tremendous toll on our relationship. Although I was experiencing depression and loss, I pushed past my anxiety and fear and decided to focus on the love and commitment that had brought us so far.

I did not have the physical energy to express much of anything emotionally or physically at that time. The aftereffects of transplant had significantly affected my sexual relationship with Cecilia. I had no desire whatsoever. In addition, we had been so busy struggling with our roles of survivor and caregiver that we had little energy left to be a loving intimate couple. So while most couples decide to get married at the cusp of a wave of physical attraction, euphoria and bliss, for us and especially me, the decision came when we were in the wave's trough. It was not that the emotion or the romantic love was not there. It was. It was simply that I lacked the physical energy to catalyze much of it.

Love, I have learned, is not merely a euphoric feeling or a burst of physical fireworks. It is a conscious act – an undercurrent of commitment, the kind of commitment I had seen from Cecilia. We decided it was time to make that commitment official. So, during a cool evening in March, we took a giant leap toward the future. Before a roaring fire at sunset, my friend and trumpeter, Linda Brown, played "Saint Elmo's Fire," heralding in a new season in our lives.

Cecilia and I were married before a small group of friends in an old ranch house south of Calgary. In a simple but elegant white dress, she was as radiant as any bride could be. I put on my best and only suit jacket, and with a small crop of fresh hair topping my head, I faced Cecilia and confidently pledged my life to her.

I recalled some lines that a friend had once given to her daughter:

Cancer is so limited…It cannot: cripple love, shatter hope, corrode faith, destroy peace, kill friendship, suppress memories, silence courage, invade the soul, steal eternal life or conquer the spirit.

– Author Unknown

"We've somehow managed to hold on to that place over the rainbow," Cecilia said to me peacefully. "We've been through a lifetime of ups and downs in just a few months. If we can keep climbing the medical mountain, we can certainly climb the marriage mountain too."

We felt joy, relief and a sense we could look forward to the future – something we had not had the luxury of doing in a long time. Cecilia was still my best friend and I hers, and considering what we had been through, that was amazing. Our marriage was a triumph of hope over adversity.

We delayed our honeymoon. We saved that treat for when my immune system was stronger and when we had been given the green light from the doctors to travel overseas. Perhaps we would go to New Zealand or Australia if we could find the money. For the time being, it was best to play it safe and stay on North American soil rather than risk contracting a foreign illness from which I might be unable to recover.

After the wedding, Cecilia and I returned to a local hotel. We were too tired to stay up much past midnight. The next morning, we slept in late and reflected on love and miracles.

CHAPTER 38

Cecilia
NEW
BEGINNINGS

Although we are creating many fresh starts, our apartment makes me feel trapped, just as I have felt trapped in my caregiver role. I have come to believe a new home will help immensely, and Alan has agreed to investigate the possibilities with me.

We start by looking at condominiums in the city, but soon realize this is not where either of us would like to live. The city now seems crowded and dirty to me, filled with pollutants. There are too many toxins.

We analyze what we need to rebuild ourselves. We ask ourselves the one important question: Where do we *really* want to live? The answer is obvious – in the mountains. We both draw energy from the mountains and feel a sense of freedom and joy when we are amongst the peaks. Alan moved to Calgary from eastern Canada over fourteen years ago to be near the Rockies. My vision board in Boston displayed photographs of mountains: clear emerald-green lakes, a log cabin, a dog, horses and fields of wildflowers. These are all the things I love and want in my life. My move to Canada brought me one step closer to that vision. Perhaps, after all we've been through, it's time.

Through a friend, we are given the name of a real estate agent in

Canmore, just a twenty-minute drive east of Banff National Park. It's a place to play that's filled with young active people like us. This is where we go to hike, bike and experience natural beauty. It has always been the center of our favorite playground.

We drive around to several locations in town, each one with a special charm. I take notes for later consideration. We look at various single-family homes in quaint little neighborhoods. There are children playing in the street and dogs barking, but these surroundings seem too much like life in the suburbs. Our last look is at a condominium complex tastefully designed to blend into the natural surroundings. There are walking paths winding through the spruce trees on either side of the street. As we pull into the driveway, I remark to the agent how quiet it is. He explains that out of the twenty-three units, there are only five full-time residents. The remaining units are recreational properties owned by weekenders.

We walk into one unit and the agent leads us up the stairwell to the top floor. Immediately, I'm struck by the incredible view provided by cathedral ceilings and expansive windows that bring the outdoors in. My heart fills with joy. I step out onto the deck that looks out over a bubbling brook. Two Mallard ducks are bobbing away in an adjoining pond. The Bow River is just a few hundred feet away and the green space between the condo and the waterway is a natural habitat for wildlife. Elk graze here year-round. Beavers build their dams in the creek, waterfowl waddle along the banks. There are no tall buildings of gray concrete staring back at me. There are no sirens and car horns. I see only snow-capped peaks touching a cobalt-blue sky. I feel open and free, surrounded by limitless possibilities for adventure. We point up at some of the summits we have attained and the ones we have yet to reach. There is a new excitement between us, just like when we first met. It tickles me to feel this way again. I take a deep breath of the cool clean mountain air and whisper to myself, "Now *this* is a place to rebuild. *This* is a place where we can heal." While the city apartment is just a temporary port from which to come and go, this is different. This could become a home. We could set down roots here. So we decide to buy.

Just as Patti Mayer performed the spiritual cleansing of Alan's hospital room, I have another extraordinary woman cleanse our new home before we move in. She walks through each room, the pungent smell of burning sage wafting behind her.

The stage is set for yet another new beginning.

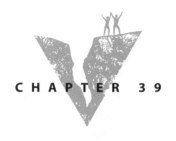

CHAPTER 39

Alan
REBIRTH

"There is far more to life than what we see."

– Patti Mayer,
From Everest to Enlightenment

A week after our wedding, we flew to California for my first speaking presentation since my illness. There, I put our immediate past aside and for sixty minutes told my Everest story. I mentioned leukemia only once – very briefly at the end. To my complete surprise, when I was finished, the audience of about five hundred rose to its feet. It was not only an affirmation of our efforts, but also a hint of greater things to come.

Cecilia and I returned home two days later. I soon fell sick with a heavy cold and nausea.

"You get sick of riding roller coasters," I wrote in my diary. "In fact, you get sick on roller coasters. I wonder if I'm ever going to be able to return to some semblance of predictability or stability at all in my life…I came home tonight and channel-surfed, wondered where my life was going again, and just a couple of days ago, I was on one of the most magnificent highs of my life. I've got to remember what it's like on the peak when I'm in the valley. That's certainly where I am today…hanging out in the apartment alone with myself, my thoughts and my fears."

I had little time to brood or recover. No sooner had we returned to the office the next day when we received an urgent call from Bernie Swain, the CEO of the Washington Speakers Bureau. He explained that a speaker they had booked for an important cancer fundraising dinner on April 6 in California had fallen sick and they needed someone to stand in as a replacement immediately. Could we do it?

Cecilia was now my sales and marketing director and a fifty percent owner of our business. She did not have to even consider the question. She just said, "No."

"You're not well," she said decisively. "You've just gotten back on stage and already we're pushing the envelope. Besides, we physically can't get from Calgary to California in time. It's out of the question."

We called Bernie back and graciously declined. He was very understanding, but also very persistent.

"I need a personal favor here from both of you," he appealed. "This is a very big group and their whole fundraising for the year hangs on this dinner. Last year they raised $4 million for the local cancer center and they do wonderful work. If there's no speaker, there's no fundraising. The speaker is the whole event. I've put Alan's name forward because I feel he's exactly the man for the job. They want to hear his cancer story."

During my convalescence, I had tried to distract myself from the boredom by beginning to incorporate some of my cancer experiences into my public speaking presentations, what I had learned, and most importantly, how others could benefit. The problem was that I was having a hard time processing an experience I was still living. It was a bit like sitting in a boat in the middle of a storm and trying to explain to others how to survive it. It was tough enough just to stay upright and afloat, let alone paddle forward.

"You need to honor your feelings," Helen MacRae had told us one day during counseling. "If the story's not yet ready to tell, it's not ready. It might never be ready. And you know what? Maybe that's okay. Some things aren't meant to be shared publicly. All of us have private lives and it's hard to find something more private than our personal health. If you choose to keep leukemia part of your private life, no one will fault you for it. Just talking about it is bound to cause you emotional discomfort, let alone trying to do it in front of thousands of people. The questions you need to ask are whether you can handle that and, more importantly, if you really want to."

Much as the creative process might be painful, I thought it might also be cathartic. I could get things out in the open. I could cleanse myself. And, if I could find the courage to speak publicly about such a personal experience, perhaps it might give others permission to open up in whatever way they felt comfortable. Cancer had a stigma attached to it. It shut in people, isolating them much as leprosy had done. The disease was so closely associated with death in many peoples' minds that the mere word evoked apprehension and fear.

I did not have such a perspective. The only way I had learned to cope with fear was to face it. If I was climbing a few thousand feet up an ice face, there was no sense ignoring my fear. I had to recognize the danger and the consequences of a mistake. But that did not mean I focused on my fear. That was a mistake just as potentially lethal as a misplaced step. I had to focus on what I needed to do to stay alive. I focused on my feet and hands, my partner, our surroundings and the weather. Mostly, I focused my mind.

So, slowly, I focused on writing. At first, it was worse than writer's block. It was writer's ice block. For hours I would sit almost motionless at the keyboard, chipping out only the odd word and a few sentences. But gradually, the ice block thawed. Frozen fragments melted into a puddle. Sentences became paragraphs and the paragraphs pages. They came pouring out of me. The process *was* painful, and some nights I cried over it, but my soul-searching was revealing the richness of what we had been through.

Not to share this treasure-trove of learnings, we concluded, would be far more painful to us in the long run than keeping our experiences bottled up. Yet the subject of cancer would have to be handled very carefully if my goal was to inspire. I chuckled to myself when I realized that public speaking was people's greatest fear and that fear of cancer was number two. Fear of death, surprisingly, was number six. I wondered where a fear of heights or the cold was on the scale. I had them like everyone else. The inner and outer Everests were directly analogous.

To that point in my recovery, however, I had believed that I would have lots of time before I would actually have to talk about cancer in a career setting. It was one thing to honor Bolek at a cancer fundraising dinner amongst friends in my home town. It was quite another to tell my story in another country to a group of strangers. Thanks to Bernie, it looked like I had to be ready now, much earlier than I had expected. And, the audience wanted to hear my cancer story.

I swallowed hard. It had only been four months since my transplant. Were they serious? So soon? I was just getting back on my feet. I was not yet prepared to pour my heart out on stage. Besides, we could not even get there in time.

"We'll send a plane," Bernie stated determinedly.

No one had ever offered to send a plane. They had sent a cab, but a plane? Bernie had to be kidding. The client was not going to cover that cost. It would easily run into the tens of thousands of dollars.

"The client won't be covering the cost," Cecilia said. "Bernie and the bureau will. He has committed to providing a speaker and obviously he has every intention of delivering one. His word is his bond."

Now we were really in a spot – and at a crossroads. If we risked traveling to an engagement and my health deteriorated further, I might end up right back in hospital. I had vowed I would never return there. In spite of the magnificent medical treatment I had received and continued to receive at Foothills, I would sooner die than go through chemotherapy again. Visions of Dr. Poon's initial diagnosis danced in my head. I could feel the darkness closing in again.

"Maybe it won't be that bad," Cecilia said suddenly. "If they send a plane to pick us up, we won't have to expend all the time and energy checking in bags, connecting through airports and risking your health in large crowds. It could keep your health risks to a minimum."

I was stunned. This was a radical about-face.

I thought of what my life would be like were it not for the Tom Baker Cancer Centre, the Special Services Building and the Foothills Medical Centre. Someone, somewhere, had found the money needed to build and operate those facilities, purchase the costly medical equipment, pay the doctors, nurses, personal care assistants and so on. I thought of patients like Rod, Andrew and Jim Cleghorn. I knew what their lives and mine would be without that funding. They would not exist.

Personally, I had a choice, but ethically and morally, did I?

"Okay," I said, throwing caution to the wind. "We'll give it a go. But if my health starts to crater, we're coming home right away. We don't want to have to explain to Dr. Russell and his entire team how we ruined all their hard work in the first four months after transplant. They wouldn't be impressed and I could hardly blame them. They're trusting us to make the right decisions. Are we?"

"Maybe we are, maybe we aren't," Cecilia wavered. "I guess only time will tell. I promise to watch you closely."

"I have no doubt you will," I reflected, knowing that was a given.

No sooner had we made the decision than I felt a wave of nausea. Within minutes, I was being sick into one of the wastebaskets at the office.

"Bad call," I thought to myself when it was over. "This is lunacy. We have made a mistake and my body just told us so."

Things got worse a few minutes later when the client called.

"Unlike some groups," the voice said, "we *want* to hear your cancer story and *only* your cancer story. Can you leave Everest out?"

Leave Everest out? The idea seemed inconceivable.

"Unfortunately, I can't leave Everest out," I ventured. "It's an integral part of how I've survived cancer so far. The skills I learned on Everest I still use on my medical mountain today. And the good news is that others can apply them too."

"I see," the client said, disappointed. "Well, all right then. Just do your best."

"Thank you," I expressed. "That's all any of us can do."

So it was a go. To succeed, Cecilia would have to do all the legwork behind the scenes while I rested and prepared once we got there. It would need to be a true team effort. If either one of us dropped the ball, we would let Bernie, the client, the cancer center and thousands of cancer patients down.

At the appointed hour, the plane arrived. We got in, and minutes later, the aircraft was airborne. In a few short hours we arrived and Cecilia went straight to work. I went straight to bed.

The promotional materials for the other speaker, a very high-profile and courageous physician who was herself a cancer survivor, were still in place when I was called to the stage the next day. The chairwoman for the event apologized for the last minute change and very graciously introduced me. I wondered if the crowd would be disappointed that this unknown presenter had been asked to substitute.

Fortunately, the audience did not seem to see it that way. The crowd was not only sympathetic to my situation, but deeply receptive to my message. I wove together my Everest adventures with my cancer climb, drawing frequent parallels, and when I was done the crowd leapt to its feet. Many of the audience members were in tears.

Cecilia rose to her feet too and applauded our collective triumph. I was so proud she could be there to see it. I thought of what courage and strength she had shown to get us there. We were out of the hospital, back on our feet and back inspiring lives. It was pretty unbelievable to experience and even more gratifying to share. It was a moment of great victory and we celebrated it together.

At that moment, I had an epiphany. To that point in my life, I had believed I had been born to climb Everest and positively affect others by talking and writing about it. Now I realized I had been born to climb Everest so I could survive cancer and help others survive, and thrive, beyond it. The next step in my life's journey had now been revealed.

Suddenly, my perspective shifted from being to knowing, yet knowing in my being what it was I had to do. I had to inspire others to climb back. I had to empower them to reach their own summits. I recalled something one of the nurses had written on Bolek's man-made mountain:

"We have been inspired to dream," Delsie Sordi wrote, "to aim high, yet keep humility in our hearts to remind us that we are but pilgrims sent with a purpose."

At last I knew my life purpose. It was not to climb Everest. Everything I had been *doing* all the years of my life was in preparation for this new raison d'être. I was being groomed for *being* in another role.

This recognition flowed over me like a cleansing shower. It was affirming – and electrifying. For the first time I truly understood my illness.

"Okay," I thought to myself as I began to shake hands and speak with audience members, "I am starting to get it now. This is all beginning to make sense. It's not about 'me.' It's about 'we.'"

CHAPTER 40

Cecilia
A CHANGE OF PLAN

At last, I have planned a long-awaited break with my two dear friends, Jan and Janet. Our time together is always filled with joy and laughter as we joke and reminisce. At the many insurance conferences we attended together, we would sit outside in the sun after long days in session, soaking up the rays and engaging in heated business discussions.

Jan and Janet are the links to my past life. Both are very accomplished businesswomen, and I revel in their successes. I can hardly wait to see them. It has been two years since we had an opportunity to get together. It will be time for me to re-energize, to talk about their lives and catch up on an industry in which I worked most of my life.

As much as I am looking forward to this time away, I am reluctant to leave. Having been by Alan's side continually for almost a year, I question if it is prudent to go. But I know I must get away. Sooner or later, we have to be apart.

I still feel a little hesitant as the flight takes off from Calgary. I take a deep breath to help steady myself. There are so many thoughts running through my mind. Will Alan be okay while I'm gone? Will I be able to relax? Or will I just be thinking about him the entire time?

Before meeting Jan and Janet in Florida, I visit my dad in New Orleans. I haven't seen him in over a year, and there are those pangs of guilt I always feel at being absent for so long. He's now in his 80s. I wonder if his appearance will have changed. Maybe he'll be a little grayer and moving a little slower – of course everything moves a little slower in New Orleans. I will have time to sleep in, walk barefoot in the grass and eat watermelon on the front porch.

It is 5 p.m. and my father and I are just sitting down to an early dinner when the phone rings. Alan's voice is on the other end.

Immediately I think, "Why is he calling? Is he all right or is he back in the hospital?" I quickly ask how he's feeling. When he says "Fine," I relax a little. He tells me about a call he just received from a producer at *The Oprah Winfrey Show*. He says he has been asked to appear in Chicago for an upcoming segment and the producer needs videotapes, background information and photographs sent overnight.

"Overnight?" I ask. "When do they want you to appear?"

"In two days," Alan says.

"Two days!" I scream. My dad shoots me a curious look.

Thoughts flash through my mind. What a great opportunity for Alan to share his story with such a large audience. How often do you get a chance like this? And then, selfishly, *what bad timing.* I want to finish visiting with my dad. I want to see my friends. I want to walk on the beach and relax.

Before I realize it, I'm saying I will call the airlines and take the next flight home.

There's a flight departing for Calgary in an hour. Frantically, I throw my clothes in my suitcase and ask Dad if he can drive me to the airport. Without hesitation, he grabs his car keys. At that point, I stop.

What am I doing? It is a forty-five-minute drive to the airport *without* rush hour traffic. There is no way I'm going to make the flight.

"What just happened?" I think. All intelligent thought process just vanished. One moment, I was having a relaxing dinner with my dad and the next I'm running for a plane.

Dad and I finish dinner. I will leave in the morning.

After dinner, I pause to collect my thoughts before making the dreaded phone calls to my friends. I feel I am letting them, and myself, down. I call Janet first. She answers in an upbeat enthusiastic voice and I tell her my situation. She laughs and says, "Do you mean we've been upstaged by Oprah?"

Next I call Jan. In her usual lighthearted fashion, she teases me until I am rolling in laughter. This makes it even harder to leave. I love these women. They are true friends.

So much for walks on the beach with girlfriends. I will have to settle for a brush with fame and a walk in the wind along the shore of Lake Michigan.

CHAPTER 41

Alan

TRIUMPH

*"You've got to aim for the horizon
and never doubt that you'll make it."*

–Mike Beedell,
Adventurer,
One Step Beyond

Further reminders of our new role in serving others now began to occur with increasing frequency. In early May, Cecilia and I appeared on *The Oprah Winfrey Show* after the producers read about my presentation at the cancer fundraiser in California in the *Los Angeles Times*. Dr. Russell asked me if I would sit on the board of the Canadian Blood and Marrow Transplant Group, an international organization responsible for promoting excellence in patient care, research and education in blood and bone marrow transplantation. Meanwhile, patients whom I had befriended during treatment now began to call upon me for advice on how to survive treatment and thrive beyond it. Some had had adult blood stem cell transplants for leukemia as I had. Others were surviving other forms of cancer. I also spoke several times to Wayde Gallant's mother, Delia, in eastern Canada. She was still struggling with her loss. It seemed to help both of us.

Slowly, thanks to consistent cardiovascular activity, proper diet, rest and the body's phenomenal healing abilities, I began to require less and less sleep, recovered more quickly after expending energy and experienced less fatigue. My muscle mass and strength began to increase. The highs and lows of the emotional and physical roller coaster I had been riding began to flatten out. There were some unexpected surprises, such as my sudden and violent reactions to foods that did not agree with my new constitution, but by now these types of incidents had become a routine part of my life. They too began to occur with less frequency. Through the clouds, the sun started to break through.

One day when I was in the Bone Marrow Transplant Clinic, a transplant patient arrived in a wheelchair pushed by his wife. He looked deathly pale. Seconds later, he fell unconscious and went into cardiac arrest right in front of me. The doctors and nurses moved swiftly to perform cardiopulmonary resuscitation, but he did not survive. He apparently had had a relapse about a year earlier and had been losing ground ever since. The incident was another clear reminder of the stakes that all transplant survivors were facing and how fortunate I was just to be alive. To watch someone die in front of you is difficult enough, but to watch him or her die after the same treatment you received hammers home the lesson of gratitude with immeasurable force. We cannot afford to take even a single moment for granted because it may be our last. We must celebrate everything we have today.

Despite these powerful reminders of how fortunate I was just to be alive, I did not always appreciate my good fortune as much as I might have. I was rarely satisfied with the speed and degree of my physical progress and I was plagued with emotional insecurities. I vacillated between hoping and planning for the future and doubting if I would actually have one. Sometimes, I was calm and confident. At other times, I was unsettled and afraid. Mixed into this melee was an unhealthy dose of guilt that I had survived while others had not. It was a hard place to be.

My fears of a relapse never went away. Every time I would get a sore throat or cold, begin to feel run down or start to show symptoms similar to those that had initially led to my diagnosis, I had flashbacks of chemotherapy, blood draws and nausea. I soon learned that although these anxieties could not be controlled, they could be managed using rational thought. Whenever I had fears of a relapse, I would counter with self-talk: "Wait a second, Alan. Has this been going on for weeks?" The answer was usually "no," in which case I would wait a few days. Usually the symptoms disappeared, often overnight. If they did not, I would call the Bone Marrow Transplant Clinic and arrange for a blood test or take any other steps to alleviate my concerns.

Beyond that, I resigned myself to fate. If my leukemia came back, it came back. If it did not, it did not. I would cross any bridges when I came to them. To live in constant fear seemed to me to be a waste of the precious energy and time I had been given. The more I looked forward, the more confident I felt. And with every passing day, that confidence increased. I could see my leukemia falling further and further into the past, and the present and future taking on an increasingly important role. By the end of June, six months after the transplant, that future was becoming clearer.

I was asked to be the closing speaker at one of the world's largest biotechnology conferences. When I finished my presentation, the three thousand or so people in attendance rose to their feet for almost a minute. I was moved close to tears, but that was only the beginning. Afterwards, Cecilia and I shook hands and signed books for more than four hours as people from many nations came by to congratulate us and share their own personal stories of trial and triumph. We knew then that there were millions of other survivors who had never had a cheering section, but who desperately needed and deserved one. Cecilia and I could become the cheerleaders.

In July, Lance Armstrong, the bicycle racer and cancer survivor, won his third Tour de France (he would go on to win more), an accomplishment that in and of itself is amazing, but against the backdrop of prior cancer treatment is absolutely astonishing. I was inspired and intrigued by this extraordinary achievement and wondered if it might still be possible for me to return to my pre-cancer level of fitness. Could my new bone marrow eventually respond with the production of a high number of strong and healthy red blood cells? If so, when, and to what degree?

The first step toward finding out was to determine my level of fitness. So I reported to the Human Performance Laboratory of the University of Calgary and climbed onto a stationary bike. Exercise physiologists Drs. David Smith and Stephen Norris, along with my endurance coach, Cal Zaryski, looked on as I was hooked up to a machine that analyzed the gases expelled in my breath. As I pedaled against an increasing resistance, blood samples were taken at periodic intervals.

When the test was complete, Dr. Smith, who had worked with many Olympic gold medalists, declared: "Congratulations, Alan. You are remarkably fit for a guy who has been through a near-death experience. However, we detect from your results that you have been exercising too hard. Try reducing your intensity and you may see improvements."

I did, and it worked. Within weeks, I noticed an increase in my energy to a level that approached that of pre-transplant. I discovered that less intense physical activity could be more healthy, more productive and best of all, more energy-producing. If this worked for me, could it work for others? This was exciting!

My goal became to return to as high a level of fitness as possible. My "blue sky" dream was to return to the level of fitness I had had prior to my last Everest expedition. Cecilia noticed that my competitive nature was becoming stronger by the month.

"It's good to see the gleam in your eye returning," she told me one day, "and the fire in your belly. Your passion is starting to come back."

For the first time in a very long while I had not only a health goal, but a physical goal, and I soon developed a training schedule to go with it. There were good training days and bad ones. The minute I walked in the door of our apartment, Cecilia could tell from the look on my face exactly what kind of a training session I had had. From her perspective, life was returning to normal.

I kept training – day after day. Sometimes I did not rest enough between sessions, or I overdid it and found myself right back on the couch again. But I did not stay there for long. As soon as I was well enough to stand, I went back at it as best I could. I had a passion to be free.

My climb back to life was not a sudden magical transformation. It took many months. There were days when I was tired and didn't want to train, but I forced myself into the gym or up the nearest hill anyway. Every time I felt the long and enticing arms of fatigue drawing me back to the couch, I added up how many hours of sleep I had had and if it was enough, I resisted the urge to acquiesce. Slowly, inch by inch, week by week, I clawed my way back.

By the time the first anniversary of my diagnosis came around on August 10, Cecilia and I had had enough of our apartment. We had come through hell and so far somehow survived, but it had put a tremendous strain on us individually and as a couple. Now that it looked like we had been given a second chance at life, it was time to make a few changes – for the better. We decided to buy our first home, downsize our business, reduce our staff, create a home office and focus on our relationship and our health. We also hoped eventually to buy a dog.

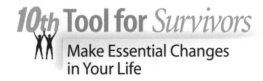

10th Tool for *Survivors*
Make Essential Changes in Your Life

The first step was to find a new place to live. After months of conscientious shopping, we found a condominium just east of Banff. It overlooked the icy waters of the Bow River and a quiet little creek complete with an adjoining duck pond. There was even a very large and healthy resident beaver we called "Brutus." Elk, deer and the odd bear regularly strolled by our back window and bald eagles, kingfishers, osprey and Canada geese frequently soared by overhead. It became our sanctuary.

Many milestones have since passed and many obstacles have been overcome. I have had the chance to speak to the manufacturers of some of the medications that helped save my life. These include GlaxoSmithKline, the manufacturer of Zofran and Wellbutrin; Amgen, the manufacturer of NEUPOGEN, which was used to stimulate the production of adult blood stem cells in Eric's blood; and Novartis, the manufacturer of Neoral, which suppressed my immune system so Eric's stem cells could establish themselves in my body. I have also been able to make several speaking presentations on behalf of the Foothills Medical Centre, the Special Services Building and the Tom Baker Cancer Centre to thank just some of the thousands of people who helped save my life. Eric and many of my friends, doctors, nurses and fellow patients, including Rod Barnes, were there.

After one presentation in October, an audience member asked: "So how come you're Superman?"

At first I did not know how to respond. After a moment to collect my thoughts, I explained, "If you think I'm Superman, you've completely missed the message in this experience. Cancer isn't just a physical challenge. It's also a mental one. We all can be Superman if we learn to train our minds to be psychological superheroes."

My eyes scanned the audience and found Rod Barnes. I asked him to stand.

"If you want to see Superman," I motioned, "he's standing right over there."

As Rod sat down, I saw him brush a tear from his eye and I knew he had been moved. As our eyes met, we both knew that our dream had come so thankfully true – we had truly met on the other side of the crevasse.

On November 15, the one year anniversary of my transplant, Cecilia sprang a surprise "Happy First Re-Birthday" party for me. My parents were visiting from eastern Canada and she had arranged for us to take them to dinner at the restaurant where we had been married the previous spring. As they had not been able to attend, it was the least we could do, she said.

Cecilia had me completely fooled until I recognized Dale's car in the parking lot. When we got inside the restaurant, I found Eric, his wife Diane,

Rita and Brian Dillabough, Dale and Cathy and a handful of others. Patti arrived later. On the tables were little bags of red jellybeans on which Cecilia had affixed copies of Bolek's "Happy Stem Cells" drawing from my transplant day calendar. Some thoughtful person had ordered beautiful corsages of white roses for Eric, Cecilia and me. A stack of very touching birthday cards magically appeared, along with a bright array of colorful balloons.

After drinks before the very fireplace where Cecilia and I had said our vows, we retired to a private room for a candlelight dinner. During dessert, I got a chance to stand up and thank each person for helping save my life. It was a pretty amazing way to mark the year we had feared I might not see, but which now promised great hope. There certainly were not many middle-aged men I knew who could remember every detail of their first birthday party. There were even fewer who could legitimately celebrate two birthdays every year. We joked that although now I could expect twice the number of gifts, for the time being at least, one of them would have to be a pull-toy. I was a 43-year-old one-year-old and proud of it. There was something quite magical about that. It was like discovering that the fountain of youth was actually inside me.

As I looked around at the shining faces of those closest to me, I marveled at miracles and the precious gift of health, family and friends. It was hard to believe they were all here – and that Cecilia and I were here with them. As everyone sang "Happy First Re-Birthday," I watched in wonder as a single sparkler candle burned its way slowly down toward the inch-thick icing on my chocolate birthday cake. We prayed the music would continue for a sweet long time to come. Every day from here on would be like the icing on that cake.

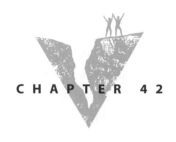

CHAPTER 42

Cecilia
A NEW CLIMBING
PARTNER

*"Wonderful new beginnings can arise
from the most tragic of events."*

– Cecilia Hobson

Ever since that exuberant day in the grass with Rita's family and her three delightful dogs, and since discovering animal-assisted therapy at the hospital, I've spent time researching the subject. I've been amazed at the material I've uncovered. There is an enormous amount of literature documenting the health benefits of working with animals, not that I really needed further convincing. Still, I've read the books anyway.

One day after our move to the mountains, Alan is reading the town newspaper and notices that a local veterinary clinic is screening animals for their pet therapy program. I want to know what's involved in the process, so I hurry over to the clinic. "I don't have a pet," I tell the examiners, "but I would like to learn more about your program. Do you mind if I sit in today?" The young girl who is assisting agrees, and introduces me to the screener, who has a kind face and a sunny disposition. She says I can observe as long as I wish.

I watch in amazement as the screener and assistant run the animals through a variety of tests to determine if any of them have the disposition to be part of the program. I am impressed with how much care and consideration is given to each animal. If there is any sign of distress or nervousness, the pair carefully comforts the pet and politely suggests to the owner that this animal might not be comfortable in pet therapy. The owners are offered pointers on how they might help their animals improve and are invited back next year for another review. I stay until every dog and cat is tested and then race home to tell Alan about it.

One Sunday morning a few weeks later, I awake with a need to take action on my ever-growing desire to own a dog. The feeling is so strong I cannot deny it any longer. I rush to the local supermarket to pick up some newspapers with classified ads. Then I drive home to begin the search for the puppy of my dreams.

I know I want a Labrador. That's the breed I have known much of my life. I know that the temperament of the Labrador will be ideal in a pet therapy dog. Sure enough, there is an ad for the sale of a litter of eleven yellow lab puppies. I immediately call but am disappointed when there is no answer and no way to leave a message. I let the phone ring twenty times. I follow up on a few other ads, but most of the animals for sale are in places too far away and I know I won't be able to make it out to see them until the following week. That seems too long to wait. I have this wild sense of urgency to find my puppy *today*.

Then the telephone rings. It's the owner of the dog with eleven puppies. Somehow she has obtained my telephone number, perhaps through divine intervention or perhaps through the wonders of telephone technology. In a kind voice, she explains that she still has three females left. She says I am welcome to come by and take a look today. I run upstairs with a big grin on my face and tell Alan I have found a puppy and we can see her right away. He's a little surprised at first but decides to go anyway just to have a look.

As soon as he sets eyes on those little balls of joy, he melts. We pick out the pup that is most gentle, sweet and loving. She comes to us when we call her and she starts nibbling on my ear. "This is the one," I say. She hasn't had her first puppy shots yet, so we reluctantly return home until we can pick her up the following Friday after her vaccinations. It's an entire week of joyful anticipation.

We take Friday afternoon off from our business to pick up our new little girl. When we arrive, she immediately runs to our feet. Alan snatches her up in his arms and gives her a big kiss. I nuzzle in and give her one too, struck with immediate puppy love. We decide to name her *Shanti*, the Hindi word for "peace." Shanti will be a catalyst for peace in our house and peace for so many others as well.

Wonderful new beginnings can arise from the most tragic of events. Shanti and I will offer our love in animal-assisted therapy. Alan and I will continue to love and heal and grow. Our new life together is taking shape. There is hope and there is joy. With a new companion tied into our rope, we will keep climbing.

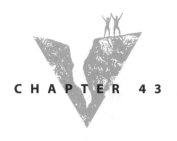

C H A P T E R   4 3

Alan
THE
FUTURE

"Medicine can work miracles, tragedy can be a teacher,
but only hope can sustain life."

– Alan Hobson

The highlight of our climb back came on New Year's Eve, a little over a year after the transplant. Before my illness, Cecilia and I had started a tradition of building a snow cave and toasting in the New Year with hot chocolate by candlelight inside it. A properly constructed snow cave is not only quiet, but also warm and remarkably comfortable. If the shelter is properly built, the temperature inside never goes below freezing. Add candles, the body heat of two adults snuggled together in toasty down sleeping bags, and the insulation created by at least two feet of snow surrounding them, and a snow cave quickly becomes a home. It can be downright cozy and surprisingly romantic.

After days of searching, we found a snowdrift deep enough in which to carve out our cave. It was two thousand feet up a mountain in southern Alberta and it took us more than twelve hours over three days to dig it. The hard windblown snow was like rock, and it took all the energy we had to carve out a space big enough for two people.

I will remember our snowshoe hike up to that cave on December 31 as long as I live. The day was glorious, cool and cloudless. The view was spectacular. A huge wide valley plunged down at our feet and the sheer ramparts of the Rockies soared skyward on all sides. The deep snow glistened in the sun's warming rays. The terrain was gently sloping and the air was filled with sweet-smelling spruce.

"Isn't this a wonderful turn of events?" Cecilia exclaimed as I helped her with her pack up the last few hundred feet to our cave. "So who's the Sherpa now?"

That night, we curled up in our snowy nest. Outside, there was not a breath of wind. The scene was absolutely still, crisp and cold.

Shortly before midnight, we crawled outside. There was a full moon. Its light bathed the snow around us in a magical shimmer that transformed night to day. The light penetrated our souls.

I thought of Dr. Poon and Dr. Russell. I thought of Rita, the nurses, housekeepers, administrators, lab technicians, radiologists, pathologists, even the parking attendants. And I thought of Dale and Cathy, Patti, Eric, Dan and James and my parents. I thought of everyone. It took a very long time.

Cecilia also paused. She took a deep breath and silently said thank you to everyone on our team. She saw Rita with the dogs and Bob McKenzie with the refrigerator, Eric making us laugh and Dale always walking in at the wrong moment. She saw my brother James' loyalty and love and all the delicious meals my mother had made that I could never eat – but that she could. All those scenes and so many more played in the theater of her mind.

Together we looked up at the moon. It was like a crystal ball. We looked into it and for the first time, our future looked bright and clear. It was no longer one day at a time. Now, we could see further – past the multitude of stars and into the limitless universe beyond. We could see ourselves biking and hiking together, sitting on a blanket in the warm summer sunshine eating endless bowls of watermelon and quietly walking hand in hand by the river outside our new home. We had ascended not just to a high point on a mountain, but to a new appreciation of life. With it came a fresh perspective and a completely new view of our experience over the previous seventeen months.

It occurred to us that life was not so much about height as it was about depth. The depth of our lives is measured in the depths of our experiences and of our relationships with others. According to an ancient proverb, "We have no enemies, we have no friends, we have only teachers." Equally, there are no good or bad experiences. There are only learning experiences. What at first appears to be a misfortune of incalculable proportion can eventually turn out to be a glistening snow-covered valley of life-enriching depth.

> *"Life is not so much about height as it is about depth."*
> – Alan Hobson

The path to this realization can be fraught with intense frustration, paralyzing fear and deep depression, yet this is the price we must pay to ultimately take hold of the jewel in an experience. It is the diamond in the darkness and we must dig long and hard under intense pressure if we hope to find it in ourselves.

We were definitely sitting on the other side of the crevasse, but now the abyss had been replaced by deeper insight. There was no end to our climb, we realized. It had nothing to do with a destination. It had everything to do with a journey. We could increase the distance from the chasm, but we could never really reach the summit. We could leave, but we could never really arrive. We could only walk our path until a new one was laid out before us.

What had started as an outward objective – to climb back and up toward a new peak – had somehow become something greater. It had proven longer and harder than any physical thing we had ever done. Like our cave, it had forced us to dig deeper than we ever had before. And it had helped us discover and define love, make new friends, celebrate family, rekindle hope, search out courage, renew determination and most of all, touch gratitude and grace. That is what we saw all around us that night: shining, shimmering grace. Somewhere out there, we knew, was truth.

The truth was that without cancer, we would not have this new appreciation and awareness of life. We might still be taking our health for granted, living in a busy city or searching for love and friendship. Without cancer, we might not be sitting here at all.

The cup was not half full or half empty. It was full, like the moon. From our little perch, we could see the light. It was everywhere.

I reached out and grasped Cecilia's mittened hand. Then I leaned over and kissed her gently on the cheek. Instantly, my breath vaporized in the night air.

"I love you," I whispered softly in her ear.

"I love you, too," she echoed as she wrapped her arms around me.

Together we shared a long passionate hug in the moonlight.

"It's been quite a journey," I reflected, gazing up at the stars.

"It sure has," she remarked serenely, "and something tells me it's far from over. We've just begun an even greater adventure – exploring the good fortune of a future."

Medicine, it seemed, could work miracles, tragedy could be a teacher, but only hope could sustain life.

> *I was once, I declare, a Stone-Age man,*
> *And I roomed in the cool of a cave;*
> *I have known, I will swear, in a new life-span*
> *The fret and the sweat of a slave:*
> *For far over all that folks hold worth,*
> *There lives and there leaps in me*
> *A love of the lowly things of earth,*
> *And a passion to be free.*
>
> – Robert Service,
> "A Rolling Stone"

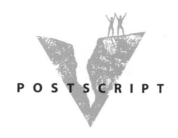

Alan

OUR NEXT EXPEDITION

"We do not just need to save lives, we need to return them."

– Alan Hobson

As this book goes to press, more than two years have passed since that enchanting evening in our snow cave. It has taken until now, about three years after my transplant, for our lives to get back to "normal." Normal, thanks to cancer, is now an anomaly. Cecilia and I do not look at a sunrise, sunset or life's simple pleasures the way we did before. We take nothing for granted. Every day is a gift and a bonus.

Incredibly, thanks to daily cardiovascular activity, I have regained one hundred percent of the fitness I had prior to my last Everest expedition. According to my research, I am now one of fewer than a dozen people ever to attain an elite level of fitness after an adult blood stem cell transplant for leukemia. My blood cell counts have returned to normal and although I still seem to react adversely to certain foods (shellfish and sharp cheeses such as feta, blue cheese, etc.), I am probably healthier now than I have been my whole life. I have been in complete remission for over four years. I have substantially reduced the number of my speaking engagements, spend far less time on the road and enjoy more time at home. Nestled in the glorious Canadian Rockies, alongside the elk, deer, beavers and eagles, Cecilia and I now live in our picture of paradise.

New Hopes and Dreams

We are so thankful to have been given back our hopes and dreams and with them, the opportunity to help others rediscover theirs. One of our dreams is to go to Everest, not to climb the Mother Goddess, but to walk at her feet imbued with a new understanding of the personal Everests we all face. Sometime after the five-year anniversary of my transplant, Cecilia and I hope to trek to base camp with a small party of friends, including some of the oncologists, nurses and other professional caregivers who have made our new life together possible. A trip to a developing country like Nepal will be an Everest in itself, the acid test of my new immune system. We will have health professionals along and we will be carrying a well-stocked medical kit.

For me, the return to the mountain will be not just a physiological marker, but a deeply meaningful emotional and spiritual experience. It will represent the shared path we all walk together, the people we meet along the way, who we are now and who we might yet become. Above all, we hope it will inspire others to climb their own inner Everests.

A New Mission

Cecilia and I have been taken with a powerful new sense of responsibility. Along with inspiring others through our experiences, we are now making concrete contributions to cancer research, treatment and recovery. We have helped spearhead a pioneering medical study into the effects of mild cardiovascular activity in reducing chronic fatigue, the single biggest challenge faced by cancer survivors.

The Rusko Test

In a meeting between Cecilia and I, two of my oncologists and three exercise physiologists, we discussed the results of a simple lying-to-standing procedure called a Rusko Test. With the help of my Polar heart rate monitor, the same device that had tipped me off to my illness, the test showed that my heart rate was stable while lying down, increased when I stood up, dropped down as I recovered from the effort and then, inexplicably, gradually rose to a point higher than when I had first stood. The exercise physiologists told us that in normal healthy people, the heart rate spikes a few seconds after standing and then eventually descends and flattens out. My test, however, more closely resembled the Rusko Test profile found in over-trained, over-tired athletes.

We wondered if this could mean something. Cancer survivors who achieve remission and whose blood test results eventually return to normal still often find themselves so weak that they cannot get out of bed, return to work or resume a meaningful life. As a result, they can become financially destitute and emotionally dysfunctional. And because there has been no clear physiological explanation for their fatigue, there has often been little that could be done to help them. This, as far as Cecilia and I can see, is not a victory. Perhaps Polar heart rate monitors and the Rusko Test might help us change this. The Rusko Test could be one of the methods of helping diagnose chronic fatigue.

Exciting New Study

After that initial meeting with the oncologists and exercise physiologists, Cecilia and I felt we had somehow pushed a snowball off the top of a mountain and all we had to do was watch as it picked up speed and size.

When elite athletes are overly fatigued, the physiologists reminded us, they do not cease all exercise. Instead, they continue to engage in physical activity but in a less strenuous way. So, that is what I did. I continued to exercise, but tried mild aerobic activity in the form of easy jogging, hiking, swimming and cycling. Within weeks, my energy level increased dramatically. That gave rise to an exciting new idea for helping exhausted cancer survivors. Christian Fibich wrote a preliminary protocol for a pilot medical study called "A Survivor Fatigue Study." We secured the donation of a dozen Polar heart rate monitors from the manufacturer, Polar Electro, and doctors, nurses and psychologists at the Tom Baker Cancer Centre started screening transplant survivors as potential participants.

This pilot study of twelve survivors was conducted jointly by the Tom Baker Cancer Centre and the University of Calgary Department of Kinesiology under the direction of Dr. Russell; exercise physiologist, Dr. David Smith; and Dr. Linda Carlson, a psychologist who works with cancer survivors. It involved a core team of about a dozen people and many others who helped with their invaluable support. Because of the severity of the treatments bone marrow and adult blood stem cell transplant survivors receive, they often experience extreme levels of fatigue. If we could find a recovery method that worked for them, perhaps it would also work for survivors of other types of cancer and cancer treatments.

Impressive Results

Each of the participants took part in mild cardiovascular activity such as walking, jogging or cycling twenty minutes a day, three days a week for three months. The key elements: their activity was *cardiovascular*; it was *consistent* (done every other day); and it was *mild* – within specific heart rate zones adjusted for each survivor based on regular performance testing done throughout the study. Now, two years into our investigation, we are thrilled to report our preliminary findings. Astonishingly, energy levels increased by an average of fifty percent to match those experienced by adults in the general population. Mood disturbances such as depression, anxiety and anger decreased by sixty-five percent, and participants reported more vigor and less difficulty with memory and decision-making.

One survivor who had only been able to work part-time on and off for eight years after a bone marrow transplant because of chronic fatigue was able to return to work full-time within a month of entering the study. Survivors were so committed to increasing their energy levels that one drove six hours a week from southern Alberta to take part in the program, while another flew six hundred miles weekly from northern Alberta (sponsored by the local airline Peace Air). Several of the study participants did not want to leave the program after their designated period of involvement. They requested access to other physical activity facilities so they could continue activity on their own. This shows the degree to which the study affected participants on a personal level. It created hope for a better life. This is the goal that now drives Cecilia and me: to instill this hope in more and more people.

The Climb Back from Cancer Protocol

We are now seeking major funding to expand the study beyond our initial twelve participants to examine the effectiveness of what we are calling *The Climb Back from Cancer Protocol* in helping three hundred survivors reduce fatigue after treatment for breast, prostate and colorectal cancer – three of the most frequently occurring cancers at the time of this writing. We also hope to create a website for the protocol. At first, the purpose of the site will be to share what the study team has learned so far, but it is to be updated as the investigation progresses and we learn more. The team wishes to continue to examine the benefits of mild aerobic activity in reducing chronic fatigue in survivors of *all* types of cancers after *all* types of treatment and eventually perhaps also in those suffering from non-cancer-related chronic fatigue, including fibromyalgia, lupus and other conditions.

The Climb Back from Cancer Foundation

Cecilia and I now have the luxury of being able to chart a bold new course in helping others. We plan to take a portion of the revenues from the sale of this and successive books in *The Climb Back from Cancer Collection*, as well as a portion of the revenues from speaking engagements and channel them into *The Climb Back from Cancer Foundation*. The Foundation's first goal will be to provide financial assistance to further prove and refine *The Climb Back from Cancer Protocol*. The Foundation's mission is simple: to turn patients into survivors and survivors into thrivers. We call every cancer patient a survivor because we believe survivorship begins at diagnosis, not discharge from hospital. We also believe that *The Climb Back from Cancer Protocol* could be used effectively from the moment of diagnosis. The sooner there are physiological, psychological and spiritual interventions (unifying the body, mind and spirit), the greater the chances of reducing mortality rates and recovery times, improving quality of life and maximizing the number of patients who return to full health. We want patients not only to survive but to "survive to thrive." We do not just need to save lives, we need to return them.

Our Ultimate Vision

Ultimately, we would like to establish *Climb Back from Cancer Centers* in fitness clubs, physiotherapy clinics, recreation centers and rehabilitation facilities across North America where survivors and caregivers could work with *Climb Back from Cancer Coaches/Consultants* during and after treatment using *The Climb Back from Cancer Protocol*. The achievement of this goal is still a long way off, but we believe it is attainable. We will start with expanding our medical study, creating *The Climb Back from Cancer Protocol* website and see where the road takes us.

Possible Future Books

The working titles for possible upcoming books in *The Climb Back from Cancer Collection* are *The 10 Tools of Triumph for Survivors, The 10 Tools of Triumph for Caregivers,* and perhaps *The Climb Back from Cancer Protocol*. These may be how-to books that explain what we believe are the key psychological and physiological skills needed by the survivor and caregiver – *The Climb Back from Cancer Team* – to survive and thrive beyond life-threatening illness. For more information on proposed and existing books you may find of interest, see the pages that follow at the end of this book.

Climb Back with Canines

Our cancer journey has been a demanding climb and a daring

adventure, but the gains have been worth the pain. Our experience has given us a much stronger appreciation for the power of the present and for each other, including our delightful yellow Labrador, *Shanti*, who has brought us great joy. She is now fully grown and weighs seventy-five pounds. Pre-training to prepare her to work in animal-assisted therapy is well underway and she is showing great promise. Cecilia hopes to develop a *Climb Back with Canines* program in which survivors incorporate the love and companionship of dogs into their daily activities. Because a dog must have regular physical activity, we see no better way to cultivate consistent physical activity in survivors than to marry it with a dog's consistent need.

Our Delayed Honeymoon

Cecilia and I continue to share our love and lives together. We finally had our honeymoon two years after my transplant when we spent four glorious weeks touring the South Island of New Zealand. "Kiwiland," as the locals call it, is without question the most geographically diverse and beautiful country we have had the privilege of visiting. Its physical attributes are surpassed only by the warmth and hospitality of its people. They impressed us with their energy, generosity and genuine love of life. We hiked, biked, backpacked, swam, snorkeled, scuba dived, river boarded (floated down a white-water river with a flutter board and fins) and caved to our hearts' content. It was a precious time to reflect on how far we had come, how much there was still yet to do and to celebrate the exciting new world of possibilities together.

Two Lives Changed

As you have seen in the previous chapters, our lives have been substantially changed by cancer. In some individuals and couples, life-threatening illness can create a desire to kick back and smell the roses. Our trip to New Zealand was certainly that, but in us and especially in me, cancer has created a considerably heightened sense of urgency. I feel a pressing need to make every second count, not only in our experiencing everything our new life has to offer, but also in our sharing of our hard-won lessons with others. Cecilia and I are together on this expedition of inspiration. We know of few other couples so fortunate, but we also know that we must each preserve our own health and, above all, our relationship together. This perspective is also one of the many gifts cancer has given us.

Expedition Inspiration

So it is that our lives have now come full circle. Somehow, we have been able to go in one end of a very long and dark tunnel and come out the other side wiser and even more passionate about life. What could have been an unrelentingly negative experience has so far turned out to be an overwhelmingly positive one. Not all cancer experiences follow this path, we know, so we have every reason to be thankful for the incredible blessings we have received and continue to receive. Each day, in fact each minute, gives us cause for celebration. We hope our good fortune will continue and we are grateful for what we have today.

We would like as many cancer patients as possible to believe that they can become survivors and as many survivors as possible to believe that they CAN and WILL climb back to life. A diagnosis of cancer is not a death sentence. It is a wake-up call – a call to action and a call to life. We can decide to try to answer that call or not. The choice is ours. Whatever we choose, the ultimate goal is to maximize our quality of life for the maximum quantity of time. The victory is in the effort, and the summit is achieved when that effort is absolute. There is no greater measure of success, or better compass with which to direct our lives. It is a higher calling – a call to a higher plane of thinking and a loftier way of living. It takes courage and focus and determination and tenacity. Most of all, it takes resolve. We must resolve to try to live – for as long as we can, as proudly as we can and as resolutely as we can. We must not give in to fear. We must seize the torch of hope.

Our next expedition is now clear. It is to gather together as much climbing rope as we can, lower it into as many crevasses as we can find, and help as many other survivors and caregivers as possible return to more fulfilled lives. Our dream is to give a hand up to anyone who is at the edge or has been to the edge and, more than anything, wants to *Climb Back!*

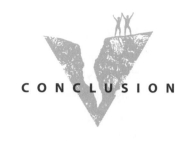

CONCLUSION

WHAT WE
LEARNED

The 10 Tools of Triumph for Survivors and Caregivers

Dear Friend,

An experience is only valuable if we can learn from it. Our cancer experience taught us a great deal. When we sat down to write a summary of the elements that contributed to our survival, we came up with a list of over two hundred items. We were overwhelmed. What became obvious was that cancer presents far more than a physical challenge. We believe the challenge is at least fifty percent psychological. Thus the mind/body/spirit connection can have a profound effect on the outcome of an illness, especially one that is described (at least at first) as "terminal." As we experienced, even among individuals of the same age, sex, diagnosis and prognosis, and who receive the same treatment, at the same facility at the same time, some survive and some do not. Is that purely physical? We do not believe it is. The power of our minds may matter more than we can possibly know. In fact, if there is a piece missing in the conventional treatment of all disease, we feel this is it. We are only addressing part of the issue.

On any expedition, there are tools we take with us in our backpacks and tools we leave behind. But in a proper pack, there are always the essentials – the items we believe will be the most important during a particular adventure. And just as there are physical tools that go into such a pack, there must also be psychological tools that go into our heads. No tool, whether physical or psychological, is effective without the knowledge and ability to use it when it is needed. When preparing for an expedition like the one cancer presents, however, we do not always know what is essential and what is not. That only comes with experience.

Thanks to our experience, we have distilled our hundreds of lessons learned into what we believe are the twenty essential psychological skills that enabled us to survive cancer and thrive beyond it. Although we cannot guarantee these tools will work for you, they did work for us. You may judge their utility, or inutility, yourself. In possible subsequent books in *The Climb Back from Cancer Collection*, we may explore how we used these skills to our advantage and how you might be able to use them too.

Here then are the psychological essentials, what we are calling *The 10 Tools of Triumph* for survivors and caregivers. Although they are numbered for easier reference, they can be used in any order. Each tool is followed by a brief description. You may notice that some of the skills for the survivor and caregiver sound similar. Because the lives of the caregiver and survivor are inextricably linked, this repetition is intended. We hope to sharpen these tools in the future. We may even decide to leave some tools behind, add more to our packs or substitute others. For now, we hope you will be able to put them to good use immediately.

As always, we send you hope, strength and courage in your own Climb Back!

Your friends and fellow climbers,

Cecilia and Alan

THE
10 Tools of Triumph™
for Survivors

1st Tool	Stay 100 Percent Present
2nd Tool	Ignore All Predictions of Doom
3rd Tool	Silence Your Mind
4th Tool	Take Charge
5th Tool	Focus All Your Energy on Getting Better
6th Tool	Decide to Be a Survivor
7th Tool	Patch into the Power of Your Personal Purpose
8th Tool	Measure Success by Effort, Not by Outcome
9th Tool	CAN/WILL® Yourself to Move
10th Tool	Make Essential Changes in Your Life

THE 10 Tools of Triumph™ for Survivors

EXPLAINED

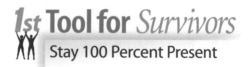

1st Tool for *Survivors*
Stay 100 Percent Present

We must not let our minds race ahead of us, imagining all manner of horrific outcomes. We must remain as calm, composed and lucid as we possibly can. That may be extremely difficult under the circumstances, but we cannot afford to waste priceless energy and time falling into fear. We may have little time left. We must make that time count – to its maximum. That means staying completely in the here and now.

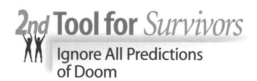

2nd Tool for *Survivors*
Ignore All Predictions of Doom

No one can predict the future. When we hear frightening news from a reputable source such as a doctor, we are conditioned to believe what we hear. But health forecasts, like all forecasts, can prove to be inaccurate. The first thing we must do is decide what we are going to believe. If we choose life, we must see the cup as half full rather than half empty. We must believe there is still the potential for survival. This is not denial, it is determination. And it is the first manifestation of a survivor's greatest single asset: hope.

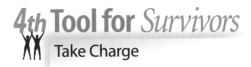

3rd Tool for *Survivors*
Silence Your Mind

Cancer treatment and recovery is emotionally and physically grueling. The psychological stress of living on the edge is intense. It is essential that we regularly escape, re-energize and rekindle our resolve. That way, we can return to the climb stronger and more effective. But because we cannot always physically change our surroundings, we need to be mentally able to change locations. Retreat into silence.

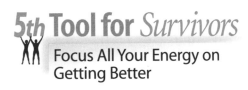

4th Tool for *Survivors*
Take Charge

Every moment that follows disappointing news offers an opportunity to take control. We can arm ourselves with valuable information, decide what treatment we wish, who is going to deliver it, how and when. We can commit to taking charge of ourselves and our care. An effective plan can lead to effective action, which can lead to an effective outcome – but only if we first think rationally and act decisively to develop that plan. Action is the greatest antidote for fear. Take it.

5th Tool for *Survivors*
Focus All Your Energy on Getting Better

It has been said that "Where focus goes, energy flows." As energy is the most precious physical resource survivors have, we must be absolutely militant in our use of it. We must dispense it with the greatest discretion. That means balancing outside commitments and personal health in a whole new way. It also means learning to temporarily say no to the needs and wants of some others and putting our needs and wants first. Our lives depend on it.

6th Tool for *Survivors*
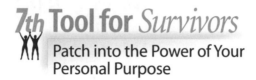
Decide to Be a Survivor

We are not cancer patients. If we are alive and living with cancer, we are survivors. We must say it and keep saying it. And we must do everything in our power to think, act and live like a survivor every day. This will not guarantee we will survive, but it will maximize our chances of doing so. To become who we are capable of becoming, we must live like we already are that person. We are survivors, period.

7th Tool for *Survivors*
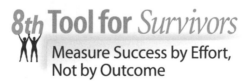
Patch into the Power of Your Personal Purpose

The German philosopher, Nietzsche, wrote that human beings can endure almost any *how* if they have a *why* for which to live. In other words, the greater our reason to live, the greater our chance of survival. The strength of our will to live is directly proportional to the strength of our personal purpose. Aside from hope, that purpose is the single greatest asset we have. It can become a beacon that guides us back from the edge. We must know why we want to live – and always remember it.

8th Tool for *Survivors*
Measure Success by Effort, Not by Outcome

Cancer is not about winning or losing. Death is not defeat. Dishonor may be. The only way to dishonor ourselves is to fail to make a one hundred percent effort. Giving it everything we have means maximizing our quality of life for whatever time we have left. Quality of life, and just as importantly, quality of effort, is more important than quantity of life. If our effort is absolute, we will be triumphant no matter what the outcome.

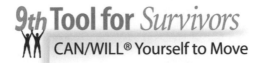

9th Tool for *Survivors*
CAN/WILL® Yourself to Move

Treatment can be physically debilitating. It can steal away our energy and leave us devoid of life and enthusiasm. But if we are to climb back, we must move. We must overcome our own inertia and sometimes, even our desire to rest. Time does not heal all wounds – we must heal our own by forcing our bodies into motion. The first step takes place in our minds.

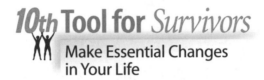

10th Tool for *Survivors*
Make Essential Changes in Your Life

Cancer is not a death sentence. It is a call to life – a wake-up call. It demands we re-examine our lives and make vital changes. If we do not, we risk returning to illness. There is no guarantee we can prevent cancer from recurring. But for whatever time we have left, we must decide what matters and what does not, what is crucial and what is optional. Change after cancer is not optional. It is essential.

THE 10 Tools of Triumph™ for Caregivers

1st Tool	Care for Yourself First
2nd Tool	Put Your Fears Aside
3rd Tool	Manage Your Mind
4th Tool	Expect the Unexpected
5th Tool	Celebrate What You Have
6th Tool	Pace Yourself for the Long Run
7th Tool	Ask for Assistance
8th Tool	Insulate Yourself Against Anger
9th Tool	Adapt to Your Changing Role
10th Tool	Support, Don't Smother

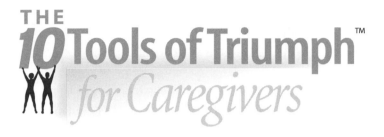

THE 10 Tools of Triumph™ for Caregivers

EXPLAINED

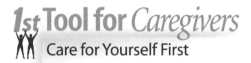

1st Tool for *Caregivers*
Care for Yourself First

If we do not care for ourselves, we cannot be there to care for our loved one. Caring for ourselves can be as simple as taking a five-minute rest break, going for a walk, making sure we are eating properly and sleeping in our own bed each night. Do it – every day.

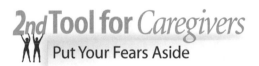

2nd Tool for *Caregivers*
Put Your Fears Aside

We will be given statistics and a prognosis that may not be encouraging. We must decide that we are going to be on the positive side of the numbers. If there is no positive side, decide we are going to be the exception. Visualize a positive outcome. Look to other survivors. Read success stories. We must surround ourselves with hope.

3rd Tool for *Caregivers*
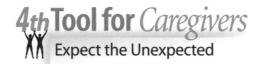
Manage Your Mind

Beware the "What ifs?" our minds can endlessly imagine. They will drain our energy and clutter our minds so we will be unable to process all the information coming at us. We must stop our minds from spinning by using whatever technique works for us – meditation, music, playing with our children, reading a book. A quiet mind is a clear mind. It is also a more productive and effective one.

4th Tool for *Caregivers*
Expect the Unexpected

Change is challenging. The new drugs, treatment methods, tests, unexpected setbacks and continuous uncertainty can wear us down. We must embrace this uncertainty and adapt to it as best we can. It is part of the experience. Concentrate only on what we can control and let everything else go.

5th Tool for *Caregivers*
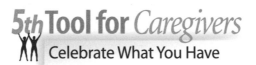
Celebrate What You Have

At the end of each day, we must think of something for which we can be grateful. It could be something as simple as a smile from a friend or a snowflake on our tongue. Whatever it is, celebrate it – and remember it.

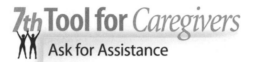

6th Tool for *Caregivers*
Pace Yourself for the Long Run

Cancer is a long-term illness. The caregiver has to conserve energy to endure the journey. If we give too much too early, we will not have enough left later. So we must find our own pace and stick to it. If we put in a very long day, we must try to make the next one shorter.

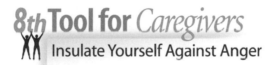

7th Tool for *Caregivers*
Ask for Assistance

Asking for help is not a sign of weakness. It is a sign of strength. It allows us to manage a demanding situation and build a support team around us. Ask for help from friends and family, but most importantly, seek psychological assistance from professionals. We cannot do it all if we want to be effective.

8th Tool for *Caregivers*
Insulate Yourself Against Anger

Anger is part of the experience – for both caregiver and survivor. If it is directed at us, remember that it can be a byproduct of medications, sleeplessness, frustration and fear. Deflect it by understanding that its true target is the illness, not us. Stand tall.

9th Tool for *Caregivers*
Adapt to Your Changing Role

Most of us define ourselves by what we do, and we are comfortable in those roles. But when our roles suddenly change, we can be thrown off balance and struggle to find our equilibrium. Our new role as caregiver must take priority.

10th Tool for *Caregivers*
Support, Don't Smother

We will want to do everything we can for our loved ones, but it is possible to do too much. If they feel they are losing their independence, resentment can build. Know when to back off. Ask them if they want help before giving them any. Allow them to do what they can for themselves. Stand strong apart and together.

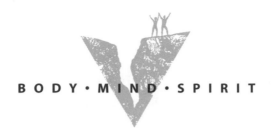

B O D Y · M I N D · S P I R I T

W H A T   W O R K E D
F O R   U S *

*While we cannot, of course, guarantee that any of these treatment methods will work for you, they worked for us. We chose a mix of western and complementary medical treatments that spanned body, mind and spirit.

BODY

- **Chemotherapy – idarubicin and cytarabine (induction and consolidation rounds) for the treatment of Acute Myeloid Leukemia (AML), M5**

  Treatment Team Leader: Dr. Man-Chiu Poon, Hematologist, Foothills Medical Centre, Calgary, Alberta, Canada

- **Conditioning for Adult Blood Stem Cell Transplant – High Dose Chemotherapy of fludarabine and busulfan**

  Treatment Team Leader: Dr. James Russell, Hematologist, Foothills Medical Centre, Calgary, Alberta, Canada

- **Allogeneic Adult Blood Stem Cell Transplant from Fully Matched Sibling Donor**

  Treatment Team Leader: Dr. James Russell, Hematologist, Foothills Medical Centre, Calgary, Alberta, Canada

ATG (anti-T-lymphocyte globulin) was given to mitigate Graft Versus Host Disease (GVHD)

- **Traditional Chinese Medicine (TCM)**

  Practitioner: Dr. Steven Aung, Edmonton, Alberta, Canada. Dr. Aung is one of very few Chinese Master Healers/M.D.s in North America. He practices medicine that integrates TCM with western medical techniques and prescribed the derivatives of Chinese herbs and plants: Golden Lu Bao Ling Zhi, Liu Wei Di Huang Wan, and something called Anticancerlin. www.aung.com; email: draung@aung.com

- **Mild Aerobic Activity** (especially hiking, biking, jogging and swimming)

  Consultants: Dr. David Smith, Exercise Physiologist, University of Calgary Department of Kinesiology, Calgary, Alberta, Canada

  Cal Zaryski, Personal Training Coach. Cal is an active triathlete (swim, bike, run), who offers online coaching to everyone, including cancer survivors. www.criticalspeed.com; email: coachcal@criticalspeed.com

  Terry Laughlin, *Total Immersion Swimming*. Terry is the world's leading coach of adult swimmers. Rather than teach you how to move your arms faster and kick your legs harder, he teaches you how to swim like a fish by reducing your body's hydrodynamic drag through the water. His program is ideal for anyone weak from treatment. He has books, videotapes and workshops. www.totalimmersion.net; email: totalswimm@aol.com

MIND

- **Counseling**

  Practitioner: Dr. Helen MacRae, Psychologist, Tom Baker Cancer Centre, Holy Cross Site, Calgary, Alberta, Canada
  Canadian Association of Psychosocial Oncology: www.capo.ca
  International Psycho-Oncology Society: www.ipos-society.org
  American Psychosocial Oncology Society: www.apos-society.org

SPIRIT

- ### Open Eye Meditation
  Raja Yoga is offered by The Brahma Kumaris World Spiritual University (BKWSU) through its thousands of spiritual centers worldwide.

  Provider: Valerie Simonson, Open Eye Meditation Instructor and Raja Yogi. www.bkwsu.com; email: calgary@bkwsu.com

- ### Reiki
  Providers: Patti Mayer, Jane Stewart, Mary Tidlund
  Eau Claire Sports Physiotherapy Clinic and The Alternative Cancer Research Foundation, Calgary, Alberta, Canada
  www.ecphysio.com or www.acrf.ca or www.iarp.org (International Association of Reiki Professionals)

- ### Acupuncture
  Provider: Patti Mayer
  Eau Claire Sports Physiotherapy Clinic,
  Calgary, Alberta, Canada
  www.ecphysio.com or www.acupuncture.com

- ### Cupping
  Provider: Patti Mayer
  Eau Claire Sports Physiotherapy Clinic,
  Calgary, Alberta, Canada
  www.ecphysio.com or www.acupuncture.com

- ### Animal-Assisted Therapy
  www.deltasociety.org or www.palspets.com

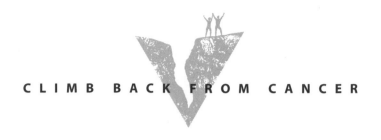

RECOMMENDED READING

There are innumerable books on the market today to assist survivors. There are far fewer to assist caregivers. Surprisingly, aside from this one, there seem to be very few aimed at helping both survivors and caregivers at the time of this writing.

The following are books of a general nature that we have read and recommend.

CANCER-RELATED

Cancer – 50 Essential Things to Do
by Greg Anderson, A Plume Book, 1999
ISBN 0-452-28074-5 (The ISBN, or International Standard Book
Numbering system is the one bookstores and libraries use to locate books)

Dancing in Limbo
by Glenna Halvorson-Boyd and Lisa K. Hunter, Jossey-Bass, 1995
ISBN 0-7879-0103-2

Every Second Counts
by Lance Armstrong with Sally Jenkins, Broadway Books, 2003
ISBN 0-385-50871-9

Getting Well Again
by Dr. Carl Simonton, M.D., Stephanie Matthews-Simonton
and James L. Creighton, Bantam Books, 1992
ISBN 0-553-28033-3

It's Not About the Bike
by Lance Armstrong with Sally Jenkins, G.P. Putnam's Sons, 2000
ISBN 0-399-14611-3

Love, Medicine and Miracles
by Dr. Bernie S. Siegel, M.D., HarperPerennial, 1998
ISBN 0-06-091983-3

NON-CANCER-RELATED

From Everest to Enlightenment – An Adventure of the Soul
by Alan Hobson, Climb Back Inc., 1999
ISBN 0-9685263-0-6 (see descriptive page that follows)

Handbook on Animal-Assisted Therapy
edited by Aubrey H. Fine, Academic Press, 2000
ISBN 0-12-256475-8

The Healing Power of Pets
by Dr. Marty Becker with Danelle Morton, Hyperion, 2002
ISBN 0-7868-6808-2

One Step Beyond – Rediscovering the Adventure Attitude
by Alan Hobson (based on the ideas of John Amatt), Climb Back Inc., 2004
ISBN 0-9685263-2-2 (see descriptive page that follows)

The Triumph of Tenacity – What It Takes To Get To The Top
(formerly titled, *The Power of Passion*)
by Alan Hobson and Jamie Clarke, Climb Back Inc., 2004
ISBN 0-9685263-3-0 (see descriptive page that follows)

You Have a Visitor
by Renee Lamm Esordi, Blue Lamm Publishing, 2000
ISBN 0-9672532-0-9

Want More?

Watch for these Proposed Books in
The Climb Back from Cancer Collection

Climb Back from Cancer
The 10 Tools of Triumph for Survivors

The 10 key psychological skills needed to cope with life-threatening illness and thrive beyond it – expanded into a practical how-to manual and workbook.

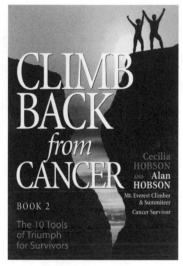

(Potential Design)

Including:

1st Tool for *Survivors*
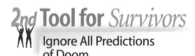 Stay 100 Percent Present

We must not allow our minds to run wild imagining all the terrible things that might befall us. We must stay in the here and now.

2nd Tool for *Survivors*
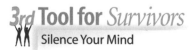 Ignore All Predictions of Doom

We can choose to believe the prognosis and die on schedule, or we can choose to try and live. We may not live longer, but we will live with greater dignity and self respect.

3rd Tool for *Survivors*
Silence Your Mind

The stress of living on the edge is intense. We need to be able to mentally retreat.

Climb Back from Cancer
The 10 Tools of Triumph for Caregivers (proposed)

The 10 key psychological skills needed by caregivers to help them cope with life-threatening illness in someone close to them. Another practical life primer.

Including:

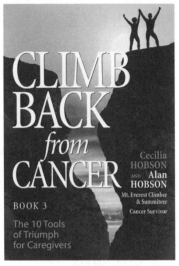

(Potential Design)

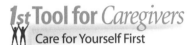
1st Tool for *Caregivers*
Care for Yourself First

To care for our loved one, we must first take care of ourselves by doing the little things to preserve our health and conserve our energy.

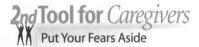
2nd Tool for *Caregivers*
Put Your Fears Aside

We must decide that we are going to be on the positive side of the statistics and surround ourselves with hope.

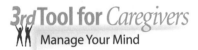
3rd Tool for *Caregivers*
Manage Your Mind

The "what ifs" can drain our energy and clutter our minds. We must learn how to calm our thoughts.

Send us an email at info@alanhobson.com and let us know which book you would like us to write next. Or, perhaps you would prefer to see a book on *The Climb Back from Cancer Protocol* or some other subject. We would like to hear from you. Deep discounts and customized editions are available on bulk orders made in advance of publication.

www.alanhobson.com

Keep Climbing!

with Alan Hobson's Other International Bestsellers…

His Gripping Ascent of Everest on his Third Attempt

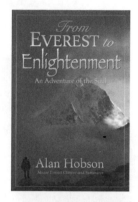

"This is a story not just about climbing a mountain, but about the mountains we are all climbing in life."

– from the Preface

His First Two Everest Expeditions

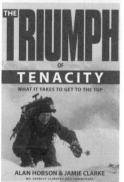

"Regardless of who we are or where we live, there is one thing we all share. We share struggle… Some days, it's a struggle to get out of bed."

– from the Introduction

Thrilling True Adventure Stories and Character Portraits

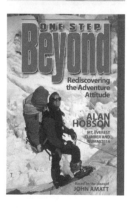

"When we run away from fear it gets bigger, but when we advance towards it, it shrinks."

– Mr. Laurie Skreslet,
First Canadian to Climb Mt. Everest

Available at www.alanhobson.com

Reach
Your Own Summit!

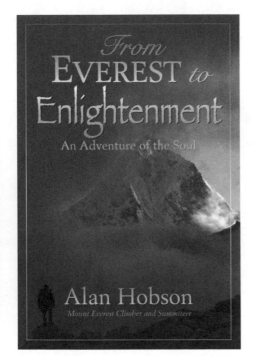

This is a book about hope, strength and courage – the stuff that is within you, the stuff that can continue to help you in your own climb back. I tell the story of my triumph at the top of the world and what it took from the depths of my soul – before my diagnosis. It took me everything it is going to take you to continue to climb your own inner Everest. After two previous expeditions that "failed" and a lifetime of preparation, I finally make it. But what I discover along the way is not what you expect.

Telling Reviews

"One of the most engaging books I have ever read…so honest, so human and so real. In a class by itself."

"Parallels to life abound. I was glued to every page."

"Truly inspiring!"

This is a Story about the Mountains We Are All Climbing in Life.

Guaranteed to Leave You Inspired!

Available at www.alanhobson.com

Take Hold of
Triumph!

Right now, right this minute. This book is the inspiring true story of my first two expeditions to Everest and what it takes to overcome adversity. Never has the triumph of tenacity and the power of personal purpose been so vital to your survival than right now. *The Triumph of Tenacity* (formerly titled, *The Power of Passion*) is the international bestseller that speaks to the heart of anyone who has ever had a dream but been blindsided by the unexpected. It's about bouncing back with more – more courage, more tenacity and more hope – the stuff that every survivor and caregiver needs.

THE TRIUMPH OF TENACITY
WHAT IT TAKES TO GET TO THE TOP

ALAN HOBSON & JAMIE CLARKE
MT. EVEREST CLIMBERS AND SUMMITEERS

Readers Rave

"Simply a fantastic read. Totally captivating."

"So breathtaking I could not put it down."

"Awesome!"

A True Tale of Persistence and Passion

Guaranteed to Leave You Breathless!

Available at www.alanhobson.com

Keep Taking that
One Step Beyond!

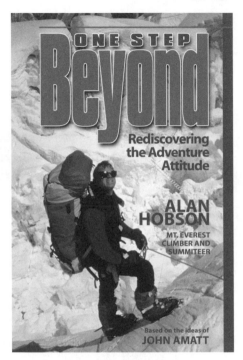

The five people in this book did. None of them had cancer, but all of them faced life-threatening adversity and won. You can too.

Five Thrilling Personal Adventure Stories and In-Depth Personality Profiles combined with the Psychological Secrets that Make the Impossible Possible!

The voices of experience speak...

- Mr. Laurie Skreslet,
  First Canadian to Climb Mt. Everest
- Sharon Wood,
  First North American
  Woman to Climb Mt. Everest
- John Hughes,
  Around-the-World Solo
  Ocean Sailor
- Mike Beedell, World Adventurer
- Mr. Laurie Dexter,
  Ultra-Endurance Athlete

High Praise from Readers

"I read a book every week or two and this book is in the top ten I have ever read."

"One of the best motivational books ever written."

"Absolutely gripping."

A Must-Read for Anyone Climbing their Own Personal Mountains

Available at www.alanhobson.com

You CAN Triumph *You* WILL!

When You Experience Alan's Speaking Presentations Live

• Riveting True Stories
• Breathtaking Color Images
• Gripping Sound and Video Recordings

"The best adventure speaker in the world."
– Bernie Swain, CEO, Washington Speakers Bureau

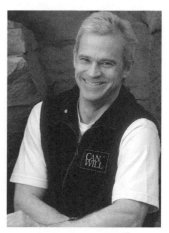

with **Alan**
HOBSON

Custom-Built for You

Alan never delivers the same speech twice. He conducts extensive personal interviews and in-depth research so he thoroughly understands each client's unique opportunities and challenges. He then seamlessly weaves the most salient points from his study into his presentation and combines them with the greatest lessons of his life experiences. The result is a one-of-a-kind presentation that has unparalleled impact and applicability.

"I have never seen, ever, in my 17 years with this firm, a speaker who learned more about us before he gave the speech. Then, he incorporated that knowledge into his presentation. It wasn't just a cursory level of understanding. It went well below the surface. He went out of his way to understand not only our industry, but our firm."

– Bob Sabelhaus, EVP, Legg Mason Wood Walker

Represented Exclusively
by the Washington
Speakers Bureau
(703) 684-0555
www.washingtonspeakers.com

Learn, Adapt, Focus and Execute with Excellence

After almost two decades of preparation and three grueling attempts, Alan finally stood atop Mt. Everest. He shows audiences how to learn from setbacks, adapt to shifting priorities and focus on executing with excellence.

Overcome the Unexpected and Seize the Tools of Triumph

Thanks to his cancer experience, Alan offers practical tools for managing the unexpected and transforming obstacles into opportunities.

For more information:
www.alanhobson.com

*Send a message of hope to someone you know
(or keep this card for yourself).*

From:

← TEAR HERE FIRST →

To:

AFFIX
POSTAGE
HERE

THE
10 Tools of Triumph™
for Caregivers

1st Tool	Care for Yourself First
2nd Tool	Put Your Fears Aside
3rd Tool	Manage Your Mind
4th Tool	Expect the Unexpected
5th Tool	Celebrate What You Have
6th Tool	Pace Yourself for the Long Run
7th Tool	Ask for Assistance
8th Tool	Insulate Yourself Against Anger
9th Tool	Adapt to Your Changing Role
10th Tool	Support, Don't Smother

TEAR HERE FIRST →

*A portion of the revenues from the sale of this book
is contributed to *The Climb Back from Cancer Foundation*
to help cancer patients, survivors and caregivers climb back to better lives.

www.alanhobson.com

THE
10 Tools of Triumph™
for Survivors

1st Tool	Stay 100 Percent Present
2nd Tool	Ignore All Predictions of Doom
3rd Tool	Silence Your Mind
4th Tool	Take Charge
5th Tool	Focus All Your Energy on Getting Better
6th Tool	Decide to Be a Survivor
7th Tool	Patch into the Power of Your Personal Purpose
8th Tool	Measure Success by Effort, Not by Outcome
9th Tool	CAN/WILL® Yourself to Move
10th Tool	Make Essential Changes in Your Life

As featured in

*Climb Back from Cancer**
A Survivor and Caregiver's Inspirational Journey

© 2004 Cecilia and Alan Hobson
Published by Climb Back Inc.
ISBN 0-9685263-1-4

CLIMB
BACK
from
CANCER

Cecilia
HOBSON
AND **Alan**
HOBSON

Mt. Everest Climber
& Summiteer

Cancer Survivor

A Survivor
and Caregiver's
Inspirational
Journey